I0113488

The Exercise Addiction Workbook

Information, Assessments, and Tools for Managing Life with a Behavioral Addiction

Ester R.A. Leutenberg and John J. Liptak, EdD

Whole Person Associates
Mental Health & Wellness Publishers
Duluth, Minnesota

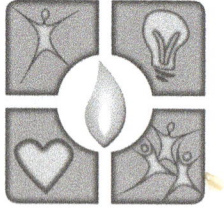

Whole Person Associates

101 West 2nd Street, Suite 203
Duluth, MN 55802-5004

800-247-6789

Books@WholePerson.com
WholePerson.com

The Exercise Addiction Workbook

Copyright ©2023 by Ester R.A. Leutenberg and John J. Liptak, EdD.
All rights reserved. The activities, assessment tools, and handouts
in this book are reproducible by the purchaser for educational
or therapeutic purposes. No other part of this book may be
reproduced or transmitted in any form by any means, electronic or
mechanical, without permission in writing from the publisher.

All efforts have been made to ensure the accuracy of the information
contained in this book as of the date published. The authors
and the publisher expressly disclaim responsibility for any adverse
effects arising from the use or application of the information
contained herein.

Printed in the United States of America

Editorial Director: Jack Kosmach
Art Director: Mathew Pawlak
Cover Design: Adam Sippola
Editor: Peg Johnson

Library of Congress Control Number: 2022942557
ISBN:978-1-57025-370-6

From the co-authors, Ester and John,
Our gratitude, thanks, and appreciation
to the following professionals:

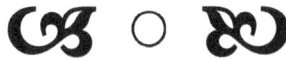

Editorial Directors – Jack Kosmach and Peg Johnson

Editor and Lifelong Teacher – Eileen Regen, MEd, CIE

Reviewers – Niki Tilicki, MA Ed

Proofreader – Jay Leutenberg, CASA

Art Director – Mathew Pawlak

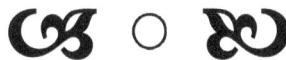

A Special Thank You
to
Whole Person Associates

for their interest in mental health issues.

Free PDF Download Available

To access your free PDF download of the assessment tools
and all of the reproducible activities in this workbook, go to:
https://WholePerson.com/store/TheExerciseAddictionWorkbook2557.html

Understanding Behavioral Addictions

There are many types of addictions. The behavioral addictions that are heard about most are substance abuse addictions. However, a behavioral addiction can be the same as a physical dependence on a substance.

> ...it is the compulsive nature of the behavior that is often indicative of a behavioral addiction, or process addiction, in an individual. The compulsion to continually engage in an activity or behavior despite the negative impact on the person's ability to remain mentally and physically healthy and functional in the home and community defines behavioral addiction. The person may find the behavior rewarding psychologically or get a "high" while engaged in the activity but may later feel guilt, remorse, or even be overwhelmed by the consequences of that continued choice. Unfortunately, as is common for all who struggle with addiction, people living with behavioral addiction cannot to stop engaging in the behavior for any length of time without treatment and intervention.

> **~ American Addiction Centers (2019)**

People are increasingly experiencing non-substance behavioral addictions and diminished control over the behavior. Behavioral addictions are no longer categorized as impulse disorders. Behavioral addictions are now viewed as true addictions, much like substance abuse.

The National Institute of Health (2010) states:

> Growing evidence suggests that behavioral addictions resemble substance addictions in many domains, including natural history, phenomenology, tolerance, comorbidity, overlapping genetic contribution, neurobiological mechanisms, and response to treatment.

> ~ Grant et al. 2010

The concept of addiction, for years adopted solely to indicate the use of psychotropic substances, is now being applied to describe a heterogeneous group of syndromes known as "behavioral addictions," "no-drug addictions," or "new addictions." Prevalence rates for such conditions, taken as a whole, are amongst the highest registered for mental disorders with social, cultural, and economic implications. Individual forms of behavioral addictions are linked by a series of psychopathological features that include repetitive, persistent, and dysfunctional behaviors, loss of control over behavior despite the negative repercussions of the latter, compulsion to satisfy the need to implement the behavior, initial well-being produced by the behavior, craving, onset of tolerance, abstinence and, ultimately, a progressive, significant impairment of overall individual functioning.

© 2023 WHOLE PERSON ASSOCIATES, 101 WEST 2ND STREET, SUITE 203, DULUTH MN 55802 • 800-247-6789 • WHOLEPERSON.COM

Why Are They Called Behavioral Addictions?

Behavioral addictions constitute any maladaptive pattern of excessive behavior that manifests in physiological, psychological, and cognitive symptoms. Hausenblas and Downs (2002) identify exercise addiction based on the following criteria that are modifications of the DSM-5 criteria for substance dependence:

- **Continuance:** continuing the behavior despite knowing that this activity is creating or exacerbating physical, psychological, or interpersonal problems.

- **Intention effects:** inability to stick to one's routine, as evidenced by exceeding the amount of time devoted to the behavior or consistently going beyond the intended amount.

- **Lack of control:** unsuccessful attempts to reduce the level of the behavior or cease it for a certain period of time.

- **Reduction in activities:** as a direct result of the behavior, social, familial, occupational, or recreational activities occur less often or are stopped.

- **Time:** a great deal of time is spent preparing for, engaging in, and recovering from the behavior.

- **Tolerance:** increasing the amount of the behavior to feel the desired effect, be it a "buzz" or a sense of accomplishment.

- **Withdrawal:** in the absence of the behavior, the person experiences adverse effects such as anxiety, irritability, restlessness, and sleep problems.

Addiction to Exercise

Exercise is excellent for everyone! However, it can be dangerous to one's health and well-being when it becomes an obsession. Some people are consumed with physical fitness and exercise. They display some or all the traits below, like those addicted to food, gambling, gaming, love and relationships, risky behavior, sex, shopping, technology, work, and substances.

TRAITS
- Obsession.
- Inability to cut back or stop.
- Dishonesty about the amount of exercise.
- Perseverance despite problems in personal relationships.
- Continuation of the behavior despite knowing it is way too much.
- Constant engagement in the behavior even though it may be causing physical harm.

Exercise causes the release of certain chemicals in the nervous system that create a sense of pleasure or reward. Because of this reaction, people become addicted to the pleasure response they gain from exercising. They then go to extreme lengths to duplicate the pleasure response from exercising.

People who feel extreme pressure to stay in shape, both self-imposed and from external sources, are at risk of developing an addiction to exercise. People who are overweight and set out on an extreme weight loss regimen may also be at risk of exercise addiction. Part of the problem arises because exercise addiction is not easy to diagnose. Most people addicted to exercise do not see anything wrong with their behavior. They believe they are doing something to take care of themselves. The constant preoccupation with exercising and working out can be a behavioral addiction that can be effectively treated using a range of cognitive and behavioral therapies.

EXERCISE ADDICTION IN THE DSM-5

Although absent from the present diagnostic guidelines, such as the World Health Organization's (2018) International Classification of Diseases (ICD) and The American Psychiatric Association's (2018) Diagnostic and Statistical Manual of Mental Disorders (DSM-5), experts have recognized that extreme exercise and workout behavior can quickly and easily become an addiction and lead to physical, occupational, social, and psychological problems. Exercise addiction is expected to be included in the next updated version of the DSM.

© 2023 WHOLE PERSON ASSOCIATES, 101 WEST 2ND STREET, SUITE 203, DULUTH MN 55802 • 800-247-6789 • WHOLEPERSON.COM

Potential Signs of Exercise Addiction

Most people do not realize that exercising can evolve from a healthy habit to a potentially harmful addiction. The main reason is that exercise releases endorphins and dopamine, the same as those released during drug use and abuse. People addicted to exercise feel reward and joy when they are engaged in working out and exercising. However, the neurotransmitters go away when they stop, and the person needs to exercise even more to trigger the same chemical releasemats.

Signs of an Exercise Addiction

The person may be ...
- Escaping life through exercise.
- Extending workouts consistently.
- Allowing other priorities to suffer.
- Worrying excessively about body image.
- Insisting on working out even when sick.
- Having uncontrollable desires to exercise.
- Ignoring a negative impact on relationships.
- Experiencing sadness if unable to exercise.
- Feeling irritable when missing a workout.
- Having marital or family relationship issues as a result of excessive exercise.
- Overtraining to the point of being sick or physically hurt.
- Finding that exercise is a serious chore and has lost its fun.
- Failing to live up to social and personal commitments.
- Increasing dependency on exercise to provide joy in life.
- Losing sleep because of exercising or thinking about exercising.
- Experiencing an inability to stick with a reduced exercise routine.
- Reducing activities in other areas of life to make time for exercise.
- Failing to devote time to other responsibilities like school or work.
- Limiting vacation spots to places with acceptable workout options.
- Undergoing withdrawal symptoms after long periods without exercise.
- Spending prolonged periods preparing for, and recovering from, exercise.

People with a mild exercise addiction may exhibit between four and five of these behaviors.
People with a moderate exercise addiction may exhibit six to seven of these behaviors.
People with a severe exercise addiction will often exhibit most or all of these behaviors.

What Constitutes an Exercise Addiction?

When considering what constitutes an exercise addiction, it is imperative to differentiate between an everyday exercise enthusiast and someone addicted to exercising. For example, are athletes or people who go to a gym to work out five days a week addicted to exercise? It is vital to recognize what represents an exercise addiction and what does not. Several aspects seem to be distinguishing factors: Does the exercise behavior become compulsive? Is the focus on working out causing serious neglect of other activities? What are the signs and length of withdrawal symptoms when the person is not engaging in exercise?

Freimuth, Moniz, and Kim (2011) suggest that there are specific phases that build upon each other in an exercise addiction:

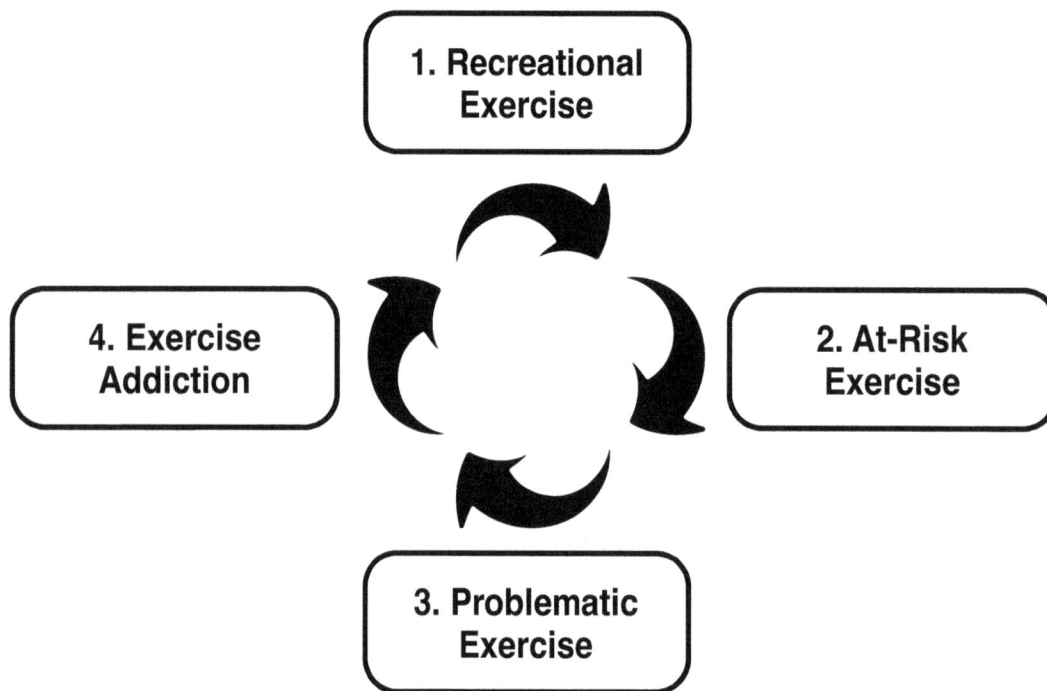

Phase One: Recreational Exercise. A person exercises primarily because it is a pleasurable and rewarding activity.

Phase Two: At-Risk Exercise. Exercise exposes the person to mood-altering effects such as the inability to manage stress and emotions or overcome anxiety.

Phase Three: Problematic Exercise. Exercise starts to become an obsession for the person. Rather than simply integrating exercise into daily life, the person often takes exercising to an extreme, lives life around the exercise routine, and will not accept anything or anyone who disrupts that routine. The person begins to experience problems functioning in daily life roles and physical difficulties associated with overexercising behavior. In addition, the person continues exercise behaviors even after reaching desired goals.

Phase Four: Exercise Addiction. The frequency and intensity of exercise continues until this behavior becomes life's main organizing principle. A person addicted to exercise will continue to work out even after feeling a sense of physical rush and gratification. The nature of addiction is paradoxical. Behaviors originally used to cope eventually make life unmanageable. As the life of an addicted person revolves around exercise, the pleasure of the behavior recedes as the primary motivation becomes avoiding withdrawal symptoms. Negative consequences in the form of impairments in daily functioning and inability to meet role obligations follow.

 © 2023 WHOLE PERSON ASSOCIATES, 101 WEST 2ND STREET, SUITE 203, DULUTH MN 55802 • 800-247-6789 • WHOLEPERSON.COM

using This Workbook

The purpose of *The Exercise Addiction* Workbook is to provide helping professionals with cognitive and behavioral assessments, tools, and exercises that can be utilized to treat the root psychological causes of exercise addiction. It is designed to help people identify and change negative, unhealthy thoughts and behaviors that may have led to exercise addiction. The activities in this workbook assist participants in identifying triggers leading to an exercise addiction and teach them ways to overcome and manage those triggers.

***The Exercise Addiction Workbook* will help participants to develop these skills:**

- Recognize an addiction problem.
- Build self-esteem with positive capabilities other than exercising.
- Become aware of recurring patterns that indicate an exercise addiction.
- Develop greater self-acceptance and the ability to change ineffective behaviors.
- Understand the triggers for preoccupation with various aspects of addictive exercise behavior.
- Reflect and become aware of behaviors that are part of the addiction.
- Learn ways to live a new life without the need to obsess about exercising.

The Exercise Addiction Workbook is a practical and flexible tool for counselors, teachers, and helping professionals working with people with exercise addiction. Depending on the role of the person using this workbook, and the specific group's or individual's needs, the modules can be used individually or as part of an integrated curriculum. The facilitator can administer an activity with a group or individual or use multiple assessments in a workshop.

Confidentiality When Completing Activity Handouts

Participants will see the words NAME CODES on some activities in the modules. Instruct participants that when writing or speaking about anyone, they need to use NAME CODES so people may preserve privacy and anonymity, allowing participants to explore their feelings without hurting anyone else's or fearing gossip, harm, or retribution. For example, a friend named Jeremy who Can Speak Spanish might be assigned a name code of **CSS** for a particular exercise. To protect others' identities, they will not use people's actual names or initials, only NAME CODES.

© 2023 WHOLE PERSON ASSOCIATES, 101 WEST 2ND STREET, SUITE 203, DULUTH MN 55802 • 800-247-6789 • WHOLEPERSON.COM

The Five Modules

The Exercise Addiction Workbook contains five modules of activity-based handouts that will help participants learn more about themselves and their addiction to exercising and working out. These modules serve as avenues for self-reflection and group experiences revolving around topics of importance in the participants' lives.

The activities in this workbook are user-friendly and varied, providing a comprehensive way to develop characteristics, skills, and attitudes for overcoming an exercise addiction.

The activities and handouts in this workbook are reproducible. Minor revisions to suit client or group needs are permitted, but the copyright statement must be retained.

Module 1: Excessive Exercise

This module helps participants explore their excessive exercise behavior by examining why they feel the need to overexercise and work out too much, use exercise to escape feelings and stress, and how they can substitute gentler forms of exercise for high-intensity exercise.

Module 2: My Exercise Story

This module helps participants explore the story of their obsession with exercise. It includes examining the form their exercise addiction takes, analyzing their current workout regimen, recognizing why they extend workouts, and identifying other issues that prompt the compulsion to exercise.

Module 3: Coping with Compulsion

This module helps participants examine the results of obsessive thoughts about their exercise behavior by looking at how to make their thinking healthier, how to control impulses to exercise, how to deal with compulsions to train, and warning signs that precede a compulsion to exercise.

Module 4: Problem Behavior

This module helps participants be more mindful of their overexercise problems by exploring missed events, abandoned activities, financial drains, neglected tasks, and the relationship issues that have resulted from excessive exercise.

Module 5: Balanced Lifestyle

This module helps participants discover how to create a balanced lifestyle by examining ways to manage excessive exercise and rest, have a peaceful sleep, journal about their exercise issues, mix up their exercise routine, and create a schedule that includes an appropriate assortment of workout times and times to rest and recuperate.

© 2023 WHOLE PERSON ASSOCIATES, 101 WEST 2ND STREET, SUITE 203, DULUTH MN 55802 • 800-247-6789 • WHOLEPERSON.COM

Different Types of Activity Handouts Included in This Workbook

A variety of materials are included in this reproducible workbook:

- **Action Plans** that assist participants in meeting the goals and objectives of treatment.

- **Assessments** that allow participants to explore their behavior. They can be used again to allow participants to track their progress.

- **Case Studies** that allow participants the opportunity to consider actual cases.

- **Drawing and Doodling** to unleash the power of the right side of the brain.

- **Educational Pages** that provide insights and tips related to the topic.

- **Group Activities** to encourage collaboration among participants.

- **Journaling activities** can help participants clarify their thoughts and feelings, thus gaining helpful self-knowledge.

- **Quotation Pages** allow participants to reflect on many powerful quotes and determine how they apply to their lives.

- **Tables** that require participants to reflect on their lives in the past, understand themselves in the present, and react more effectively in the future.

References

American Addiction Centers (2019). *Behavioral Addictions.*
https://americanaddictioncenters.org/behavioral-addictions

American Psychiatric Association (2018). *Diagnostic and Statistical Manual of Mental Disorders.* (DSM–5),
https://www.psychiatry.org/psychiatrists/practice/dsm

Downs, D.S. & Hausenblas, H.A. (2002). How Much is Too Much? Development and Validation of the Exercise Dependence Scale. *Psychology and Health* 17:4, 387-404, DOI: 10.1080/0887044022000004894

Freimuth, M., Kim, S.R., & Moniz, S. (2011). Clarifying Exercise Addiction: Differential Diagnosis, Co-occurring Disorders, and Phases of Addiction. *International Journal of Research in Public Health.* October 2011; 8(10): 4069–4081. DOI

National Institute of Health (2010). Introduction to B*ehavioral Addictions.*
https://www.ncbi.nlm.nih.gov/pmc/articles/PMC3164585

Table of Contents

(Continued on page xiii)

Table of Contents

(Continued on page xiv)

Table of Contents

© 2023 WHOLE PERSON ASSOCIATES, 101 WEST 2ND STREET, SUITE 203, DULUTH MN 55802 • 800-247-6789 • WHOLEPERSON.COM

Exercise

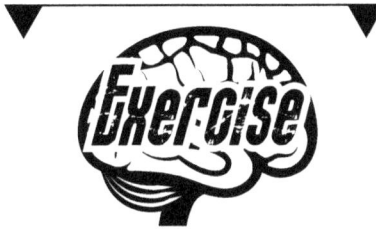

Excessive Exercise

Name _____

Date _____

© 2023 WHOLE PERSON ASSOCIATES, 101 WEST 2ND STREET, SUITE 203, DULUTH MN 55802 • 800-247-6789 • WHOLEPERSON.COM

© 2023 WHOLE PERSON ASSOCIATES, 101 WEST 2ND STREET, SUITE 203, DULUTH MN 55802 · 800-247-6789 · WHOLEPERSON.COM

Excessive Exercise Assessment
Introduction and Directions

People who are addicted to exercise often demonstrate three distinct excessive exercise regimens:

1. **OBLIGATORY EXERCISE:** People feel compelled to exercise beyond the point of benefitting their bodies. They will participate in athletic activities regardless of pain, injury, and illness. They try to arrange their lives to maximize workout time.
2. **EXERCISE BULIMIA:** People have binge eating sessions followed by periods of high-intensity exercise.
3. **BODY DYSMORPHIA:** People are obsessed with parts of their body and perceive them to be different or odd. They will create highly regimented routines to improve their perception of the "flawed" body part.

The *Excessive Exercise Assessment* will assist in exploring the above three regimens. The assessment contains 24 statements about workout and exercise behaviors.

Read each of the statements and decide whether it describes you or not. If it describes you, circle the number under the TRUE column. If the statement does not describe you, circle the number under the FALSE column.

In the following example, the circled 2 indicates that the person completing this assessment believes that the statement is true for them:

	TRUE	FALSE
When it comes to exercising and working out …		
I feel compelled to exercise	(2)	1
I exercise beyond the point of benefit	(2)	1

This is not a test. Since there are no right or wrong answers, do not spend too much time thinking about your answers. Be sure to respond to every statement. The purpose of this assessment is for YOU to learn more about YOU and your exercise habits.

BE HONEST!

If you choose, no one else needs to see the results.

(Turn to the next page and begin.)

Excessive Exercise Assessment

Name _____ Date _____

This will only be accurate if you respond honestly. No one else needs to see this if you choose.

When it comes to exercising and working out ...

	TRUE	FALSE
I feel compelled to exercise	2	1
I exercise beyond the point of benefit	2	1
I insist on exercising even if I'm in pain	2	1
I have arranged my life around my exercise regimen	2	1
I feel obligated to exercise even if I am sick	2	1
I skip other necessary obligations to maximize my workout time	2	1
I avoid other important activities to workout	2	1
I believe exercise is the most important thing in my life	2	1

OBLIGATORY EXERCISE TOTAL = _____

When it comes to exercising and working out ...

	TRUE	FALSE
I forget to fuel my body with water or food	2	1
I don't give my body adequate rest or water between workouts	2	1
I would rather exercise than spend time with family	2	1
I consider myself a compulsive exerciser	2	1
I define my self-worth by the amount I exercise	2	1
I excessively exercise because I am an amazing athlete	2	1
I do not sleep well when I get overly tired from exercising	2	1
I would rather workout than be with friends	2	1

EXERCISE BULIMIA TOTAL = _____

When it comes to exercising and working out ...

	TRUE	FALSE
I constantly think about every possible flaw in my appearance	2	1
I spend a lot of time looking at my body in the mirror	2	1
I am scared that I will become fat	2	1
I compare my body to anyone I see	2	1
I feel like I have an abnormality that makes me unattractive	2	1
I am preoccupied by my appearance	2	1
I already had or want cosmetic surgeries to look better	2	1
I think that others are always looking at me	2	1

BODY DYSMORPHIA TOTAL = _____

Go to the next page for scoring assessment results, profile interpretation, and individual description.

© 2023 WHOLE PERSON ASSOCIATES, 101 WEST 2ND STREET, SUITE 203, DULUTH MN 55802 • 800-247-6789 • WHOLEPERSON.COM

Excessive Exercise Assessment

Scoring and Profile Interpretation

This assessment measures your tendency to work out and exercise excessively.

For each of the items in the three sections on the previous page, count the scores you circled. Put each of those totals on the TOTAL spot at the end of each section. Then, transfer your totals to the space below:

Obligatory Exercise TOTAL = _____

Exercise Bulimia TOTAL = _____

Body Dysmorphia TOTAL = _____

Assessment Profile Interpretation

The *Excessive Exercise Assessment* measures the impact of your exercising behavior on your life. Even one TRUE score can suggest you are experiencing issues due to excessive exercise. The HIGHER your score the more you need to be concerned about how you work out and exercise.

Enter your scores on the appropriate lines below.

Obligatory Exercise Total: Your tendency to be compelled to exercise beyond the point of having a benefit.

8 = Low	12 = Moderate	16 = High

Exercise Bulimia Total: Your tendency to binge eat followed by periods of high-intensity exercise.

8 = Low	12 = Moderate	16 = High

Body Dysmorphia Total: Your tendency to create highly regimented routines to improve your perception of a "flawed" body part.

8 = Low	12 = Moderate	16 = High

Missing Workouts

When people have an addiction to exercise, they often experience a variety of negative emotions when they cannot work out. They may feel irritable, sad, anxious, angry, disgusted, grumpy, over-critical, annoyed, depressed, etc.

Below, explore the feelings you have experienced when you missed a workout.

When I Missed a Workout	I Felt	This is What Occurred
Example: I could not work out on Saturday because I had a family obligation.	Furious and restless.	I got into a huge argument with my partner.

If you become agitated or uncomfortable after missing a workout, even after you have had a long string of workouts over several days, it could be a sign of exercise addiction.

© 2023 WHOLE PERSON ASSOCIATES, 101 WEST 2ND STREET, SUITE 203, DULUTH MN 55802 • 800-247-6789 • WHOLEPERSON.COM

Workout Warrior

Are you one of those who work out when you are sick, injured, or exhausted? People who have an addiction to exercise push themselves through a pulled muscle, the flu, a stress fracture, etc., failing to rest when it's clearly needed. This is unfair to one's body!

What are the times you exercised when you were sick, injured, or exhausted?

A Time I Exercised Even Though I Wasn't Feeling Well	Why I Exercised	Outcome
Example: I had the flu and was coughing, sneezing, hurting, and feeling miserable.	*I didn't think it would matter, and I thought it would make me feel better.*	*It got worse, and then I had pneumonia. Others in the gym caught my flu!*

I'm addicted to exercising, and I have to do something every day.
~ Arnold Schwarzenegger

What type of exercise do you feel you have to do every day?

_____

_____

_____

I Must Work Out

Some people who are addicted to exercise feel that they MUST exercise. They feel compelled to work out and lack the control to refrain from exercise at certain times.

Respond to the following sentence starters about your need to work out.

I must work out, or _____

_____

_____

If I don't work out, I feel _____

_____

_____

If I don't work out, (USE NAME CODE) _____ **will say** _____

_____

_____

If I miss a workout, my body _____

_____

_____

If I miss a workout, my mind _____

_____

_____

If I must cut short my workout, I _____

_____

_____

© 2023 WHOLE PERSON ASSOCIATES, 101 WEST 2ND STREET, SUITE 203, DULUTH MN 55802 • 800-247-6789 • WHOLEPERSON.COM

Is Exercise an Escape Mechanism?

For people addicted to exercise, the workout process may become an escape from life's stressors, though they might not realize it. Exercise can be a way to escape from the stressors one encounters at work, home, relationships, communities, etc.

What types of situations might you be escaping by exercising?
Write, draw, or doodle them below.

Work	Home

Relationships	My Community

Escaping My Emotions (Part 1)

People who work out and exercise to excess may not even realize that they are trying to escape the challenging emotions they are experiencing. It is essential to confront these uncomfortable emotions in ways that do not include excessive exercise.

Exercise may seem to work in the short term but does not address the underlying emotional challenges. It is healthier to address the issue at hand rather than trying to escape the emotions.

Below, identify an emotion and situation you try to escape through exercise.

An Emotion and Situation I Try to Escape	How I Exercise/Workout	What Could I Do Instead?
Example: I am frustrated because my boss expects too much of me in the time I have.		*Ask to speak with the boss privately and talk about my concerns and suggestions.*

Respond to these questions when reflecting on the emotion you listed above:

What about this situation makes me emotional? _____

_____

Does the intensity of my feelings match the situation? _____

_____

Do I have feelings that I need to pay attention to? _____

_____

What interpretations or judgments am I making about this event? _____

_____

What are my other options for expressing my feelings? _____

_____

What are some ways to express these emotions without exercising? _____

_____

What are the consequences of using exercise to mask my emotions? _____

_____

Who is a trusted person who can help me process my emotions? _____

_____

Why do I turn to exercise rather than other people to process my emotions? _____

_____

What would happen if I did not exercise to mask my emotions? _____

_____

© 2023 WHOLE PERSON ASSOCIATES, 101 WEST 2ND STREET, SUITE 203, DULUTH MN 55802 • 800-247-6789 • WHOLEPERSON.COM

Escaping My Emotions (Part 2)

The purpose of engaging in compulsive behavior like exercising is to decrease internal emotional pain and internal anxiety. You can benefit by identifying and understanding those feelings and their triggers.

The following steps will help you manage your emotions rather than trying to escape them by working out. Think about a situation that triggers negative emotions in you. What is that situation?

STEP 1: Become aware of your emotions.
Could you recognize your emotions in that situation? Name the emotions you have. Are you feeling nervous? Depressed? Embarrassed? What emotions did you feel in this situation?

_____

_____

_____

STEP 2: Identify any emotional triggers.
What triggers your emotions (people, things, situations) that prompt you to feel a certain way?

_____

_____

_____

STEP 3: Solve problems rather than focusing on negative emotions.
Negative thoughts are often at the root of many of your feelings. Negative thoughts can also prompt negative emotions. For example, if you keep thinking, "I hate my job," you will feel frustrated and sad. When this occurs, you run a mile. However, if you spend your time and energy searching for a job which you would like better, that would be a more productive solution than excessive exercise. What are some solutions you can apply to your triggers?

_____

_____

_____

> All emotions are pure which gather you and lift you up; that emotion is
> impure which seizes only one side of your being and so distorts you.
> **~ Rainer Maria Rilke**

Why I Want to Slow Down

People with an exercise addiction do not stop excessive exercise immediately. They do it slowly. They remember what happens if they do not cut back. They also remember what they are doing to their bodies, minds, lives, relationships, etc., when they exercise too much.

Below, identify how you can start slowing down your exercise regimen.

Ways I Can Slow Down	What Will Happen if I Don't Slow Down	How Am I Affected By Not Slowing Down
Example: Limit my workouts to three days a week.	*I will have physical problems; my family will be upset, etc.*	*I am starting to experience joint damage, relationship issues, etc.*

- -

CUT THIS OUT AND POST IT ON YOUR BATHROOM MIRROR!

Ways to slow down:
- Keep a timer. Watch the time and stick to specific time limits.
- Exercise with a friend who can remind you to stop the exercise session.
- Join exercise groups that meet three times per week and limit other exercise sessions.
- Pick several favorite songs and stop when they are finished playing.
- Substitute less intense workouts. For example, yoga instead of running.
- Find a hobby you can engage in when you feel the compulsion to work out excessively.

© 2023 WHOLE PERSON ASSOCIATES, 101 WEST 2ND STREET, SUITE 203, DULUTH MN 55802 • 800-247-6789 • WHOLEPERSON.COM

Exercise Substitutions

People who exercise excessively often feel they must engage in the most high-intensity workout possible. A great way to break the addiction to exercise is to replace a high-intensity workout with a different (low-intensity) exercise. For example, if you run, you could try walking instead. If you are addicted to long weight-lifting sessions, try yoga instead. Trying new things gets you out of your routine and is less harmful to your body.

Below, identify some substitutions you can make in the forms of exercise you engage in.

Current exercise activities:

Example: running ten miles a day.

_____

_____

_____

_____

_____

_____

_____

_____

Healthier exercise activities:

Example: playing and running with my dog.

_____

_____

_____

_____

_____

_____

_____

_____

Perfectionism

People with an exercise addiction often have a body image they cannot compromise. It may be an unrealistic body image or a fixed idea of what their shape and weight are supposed to be. People who work out excessively often try to attain the "perfect" body.

Below, draw or describe your current body and your ideal shapes and weight. Then, state the reasons why you don't like your current body and why you want to achieve your ideal body.

My Current Body Image and Weight	My Ideal Body Image and Weight

My Negative Views of My Current Body	Why I Want to Achieve My Ideal Body
1.	1.
2.	2.
3.	3.
4.	4.
5.	5.
6.	6.
7.	7.

© 2023 WHOLE PERSON ASSOCIATES, 101 WEST 2ND STREET, SUITE 203, DULUTH MN 55802 • 800-247-6789 • WHOLEPERSON.COM

Alternatives to Exercise

People who exercise excessively do not see a way to compromise their exercise routines and cannot imagine an alternative to working out. It is vital to identify positive behaviors that will function to ensure the body and cardiovascular system stay healthy.

Below, explore your current involvement in activities (other than exercising) during your spare time. Then, explore your possible participation in new activities (other than exercising).

My Spare Time Activities Now (USE NAME CODES)	When I Do This Activity Rather Than Exercising	How the Activity Helps Me
Example: *Go to the movies with MFJ.*	*Once a month.*	*It helps me keep MFJ as a friend who complains that we never get together.*

My Spare Time Activities I Could Do	When I Can Do This Activity Rather Than Exercising	How the Activity Will Help Me
Example: *Join a community theater group.*	*They meet every Thursday night and more often when rehearsals begin.*	*I love acting and singing and will reunite with people I haven't seen for a long time.*

TIPS:
- Attempt to balance exercise with other leisure activities.
- Find activities that keep the body moving (dancing, kayaking, playing with pets).

Narcissism

Narcissism: The pursuit of gratification from vanity or egotistic admiration of one's idealized self-image and attributes, including self-flattery and perfectionism.

People addicted to exercise are sometimes narcissistic in their approach to life. They will keep looking at themselves in mirrors, enjoy the attention they get from others, and love it when others say how good they look. In what ways are you narcissistic?

Describe some of the ways you tend to be narcissistic in the circles below.

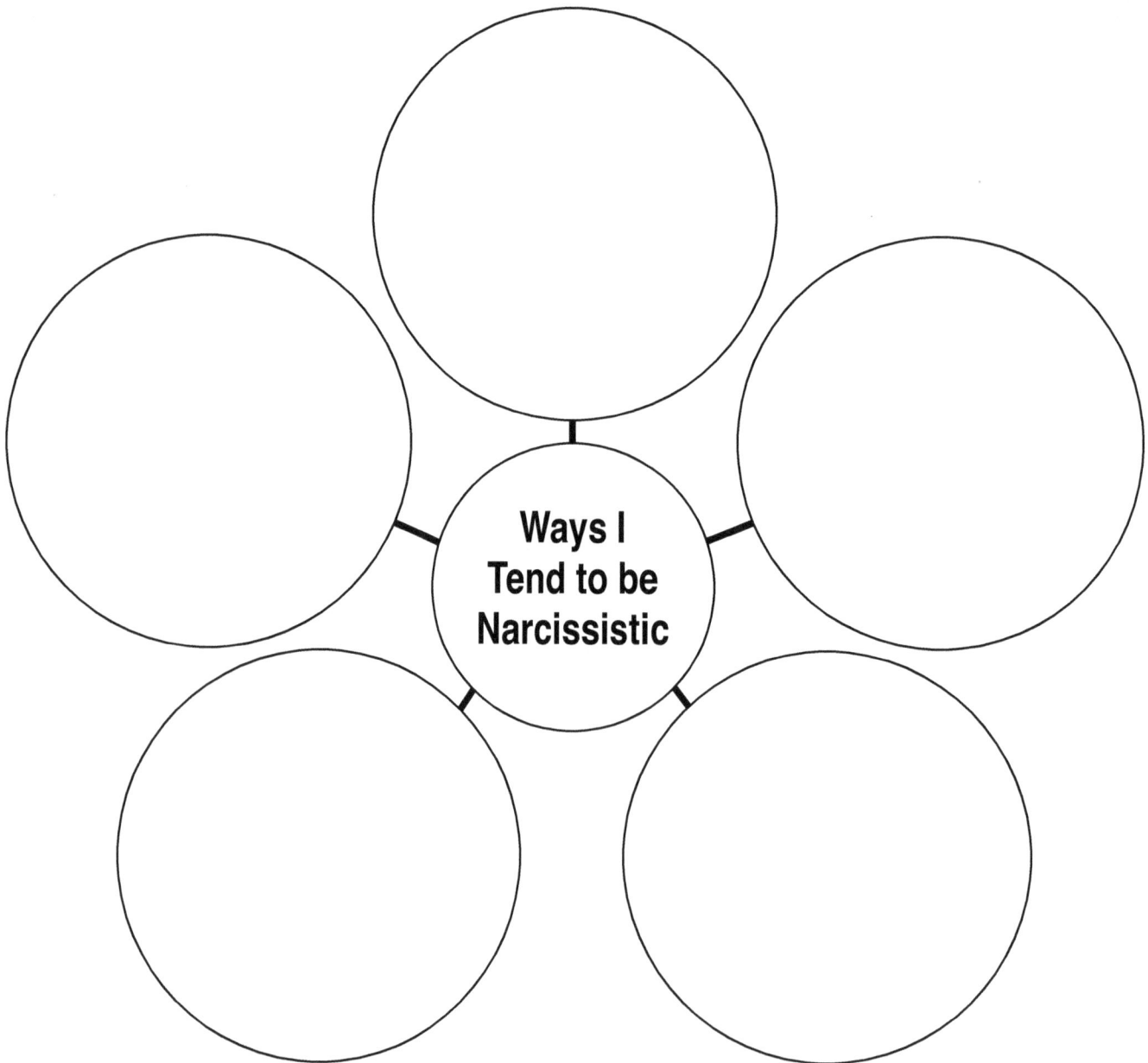

Ways I Tend to be Narcissistic

The fact is, for years, I had been trapped in a certain narcissism
and a desire to have a certain body and look sexy.
~ David Harbour

© 2023 WHOLE PERSON ASSOCIATES, 101 WEST 2ND STREET, SUITE 203, DULUTH MN 55802 • 800-247-6789 • WHOLEPERSON.COM

Exercise Bulimia

Exercise bulimia is an extreme, pathologic exercise behavior. It has some characteristics similar to bulimia nervosa. Bulimia nervosa is an eating disorder that generally involves binge eating followed by purging. Purging means ridding your body of ingested food by self-induced vomiting or diarrhea. A person with exercise bulimia doesn't purge. They overexercise to burn fat and calories instead.

People who experience exercise bulimia often have binge eating sessions followed by periods of high-intensity exercise.

Below, identify the ways you binge eat and then exercise.
Identify what you eat, how you exercise to work off the calories, and the results.

Binge Eating Session	My Exercise Workout	Results
Example: I ate a gallon of chocolate ice cream in one sitting!	*I ran five miles to work off the calories and carbohydrates of the ice cream.*	*I was late for my appointment with my customer.*

Do You Value Yourself?

If you engage in excessive exercise, you probably value yourself in terms of physical fitness and appearance, achievement, and physical performance. Do you value yourself in terms of inner qualities such as empathy, a sense of duty, the courage of your convictions, truthfulness, kindness, character, etc.?

In each of the hexagons, write about inner qualities you possess that you value.

Inner Qualities I Value

© 2023 WHOLE PERSON ASSOCIATES, 101 WEST 2ND STREET, SUITE 203, DULUTH MN 55802 • 800-247-6789 • WHOLEPERSON.COM

How I Perceive My Body

People with an exercise addiction often react to the unique ways they perceive their bodies.

On the line under each reaction, place an X on the continuum based on how you see yourself. On the dotted line below, write how you exercise to overcome it. **BE HONEST!**

I am preoccupied with flaws in my appearance.

0 (Not True)   5 (Somewhat True)   10 (TRUE)

I am always trying to overcome flaws in my body by exercising.

0 (Not True)   5 (Somewhat True)   10 (TRUE)

I seek reassurance from others about my appearance.

0 (Not True)   5 (Somewhat True)   10 (TRUE)

I avoid social situations because of my appearance.

0 (Not True)   5 (Somewhat True)   10 (TRUE)

I desperately want to have a perfect body.

0 (Not True)   5 (Somewhat True)   10 (TRUE)

The higher your score on each of the lines above, the more of a body dysmorphia problem you have in those aspects. Areas where you scored low suggest that you are not experiencing many signs of body dysmorphia in those areas.

Will your life change if you overcome your addiction to exercise?.

0 (Not Much)   5 (A Little)   10 (A Great Deal)

Do you want to change your current exercise habits?.

0 (Not Much)   5 (A Little)   10 (A Great Deal)

Experiencing Joy

If you feel like the only time you are happy or experience joy is when you are exercising, the chances are that you may have an exercise addiction.

If happiness and joy are solely dictated by the outcome of your latest workout, how your body looks that day, or how fit you currently perceive yourself to be, you need to explore other ways you can find happiness and joy.

Respond to the following questions about how you can find joy and happiness in life.

I can find joy and happiness with my family members by ...

_____

_____

I can find joy and happiness with friends by ...

_____

_____

I can find joy and happiness with hobbies such as ...

_____

_____

I can find joy and happiness hanging out with pets/animals by ...

_____

_____

I can find joy and happiness volunteering my time with ...

_____

_____

I can find joy and happiness at work by ...

_____

_____

© 2023 WHOLE PERSON ASSOCIATES, 101 WEST 2ND STREET, SUITE 203, DULUTH MN 55802 • 800-247-6789 • WHOLEPERSON.COM

Reward Yourself

Reward yourself when you successfully limit your exercise time!

People who reward themselves are more likely to limit their exercise time. The challenge is to decide what rewards would motivate you to reach your goal. A reward needs to be something that will give you the incentive to achieve. It needs to be within your budget and something you'll be excited about. If you are rewarding yourself with a purchase, be sure it is something you wouldn't ordinarily buy or do.

Brainstorm some possible rewards and record them below.

Rewards that would be meaningful to me _____

Small rewards I could give myself _____

Large rewards I could give myself _____

Things that would not cost money and would be fun _____

Rewards that I can afford and would be fun _____

Rewards that I can experience alone _____

Rewards I can do with people who support me _____

Tracking Your Goals

My Current Exercise Time	My Goal to Limit Exercise Time	My Progress
Example: I exercise 7 days per week, 2 hours per day.	I will limit my exercise to 4 days per week, 2 hours per day for 2 months.	I achieved my goal! I'm spending more time with my family, feel healthier, and will continue with this regimen.

Rewards help you pay attention to your triumphs, not your setbacks. Rewards will create good feelings and propel you to want to work harder to reach your goals. Whenever you have completed or achieved one of your goals, treat yourself to one of the items on your list.

Quotes about Excessive Exercise

On the lines that follow each of the quotes, describe what the quote means to you and how it applies to YOUR life.

Exercise is like an addiction. Once you're in it, you feel like your body needs it.
~ Elsa Pataky

_____

Joy, feeling one's own value, being appreciated and loved by others, feeling useful and capable of production are all factors of enormous value for the human soul.
~ Maria Montessori

_____

Healthy body image is not something that you're going to learn from fashion magazines.
~ Erin Heatherton

_____

Many people think of perfectionism as striving to be your best, but it is not about self-improvement; it's about earning approval and acceptance.
~ Brene Brown

_____

There's a certain addiction to sweat, for sure. I'm not the same person without it. If I don't get my hour of exercise in every day, then I'm not the person that I want to be.
~ Ryan Kwanten

_____

Which quote especially speaks to you and your relationship to excessive exercise? Why?

_____

_____

_____

_____

_____

_____

© 2023 WHOLE PERSON ASSOCIATES, 101 WEST 2ND STREET, SUITE 203, DULUTH MN 55802 • 800-247-6789 • WHOLEPERSON.COM

Exercise

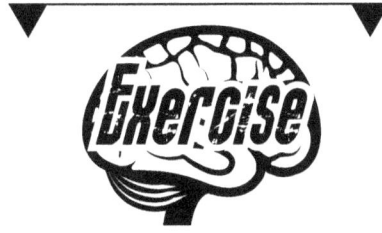

My Exercise Story

Name _____

Date _____

© 2023 WHOLE PERSON ASSOCIATES, 101 WEST 2ND STREET, SUITE 203, DULUTH MN 55802 • 800-247-6789 • WHOLEPERSON.COM

© 2023 WHOLE PERSON ASSOCIATES, 101 WEST 2ND STREET, SUITE 203, DULUTH MN 55802 • 800-247-6789 • WHOLEPERSON.COM

My Exercise Story Assessment
Introduction and Directions

Everyone has a story with a beginning, middle, and end to share the important factors that makeup who they are. People addicted to exercise have a story about their workouts and exercise behavior.

The *My Exercise Story Assessment* contains 20 statements related to working out and exercise behavior. It can help you gauge your exercise addiction risk level. The only way to be sure is to be very honest when completing the assessment.

Read each statement and decide whether it describes you. If it describes you, circle the number in the TRUE column next to that item. If the statement does not describe you, circle the number in the NOT TRUE column next to that item.

In the following example, the circled 2 indicates that the person completing this assessment believes that the statement is true for them:

	TRUE	NOT TRUE
When it comes to exercising ...		
I feel a buzz after exercising	(2)	1
I am miserable when I miss a workout	(2)	1

This is not a test. Since there are no right or wrong answers, do not spend too much time thinking about them. Be sure to respond to every statement.

BE HONEST!

If you choose, no one else needs to see the results.

(Turn to the next page and begin.)

My Exercise Story Assessment

Name _____ Date _____

This will only be accurate if you respond honestly. No one else needs to see this if you choose.

	TRUE	NOT TRUE

When it comes to exercising ...

I feel a buzz after exercising 2 1

I am miserable when I miss a workout 2 1

I experience withdrawal symptoms if I don't exercise. 2 1

I often have an uncontrollable desire to exercise 2 1

I do not concern myself about anything else when I exercise 2 1

I insist on working out even when I'm sick 2 1

I worry excessively about how my body looks 2 1

I have had failed relationships because of my exercising. 2 1

I think about exercising all the time 2 1

I am only really satisfied with myself when I'm exercising 2 1

I escape from stress by working out. 2 1

I train to the point that I hurt my body 2 1

I keep extending the amount of time I work out 2 1

I feel like my work is suffering because of my workout schedule. 2 1

I have a difficult time reducing my exercise regimen. 2 1

I am grouchy if I cannot work out 2 1

I go on vacations and work out rather than see the sights. 2 1

I don't allow enough recovery time before exercising again. 2 1

I wish I could exercise more than I do now 2 1

I exercise because I hate the way my body looks. 2 1

TOTAL = _____

*Go to the next page for scoring assessment results,
profile interpretation, and individual description.*

© 2023 WHOLE PERSON ASSOCIATES, 101 WEST 2ND STREET, SUITE 203, DULUTH MN 55802 • 800-247-6789 • WHOLEPERSON.COM

My Exercise Story Assessment

Descriptions and Profile Interpretation

The assessment you just completed is designed to measure your awareness of the impact of your compulsive exercise behavior.

For each of the items on the previous page, count the scores you circled. Transfer that total to the line marked TOTAL at the end of the section.

My Exercise Story TOTAL = _____

Now, mark your score to the continuum below.

20 = Low	30 = Moderate	40 = High

Assessment Profile Interpretation

By circling even one TRUE answer, you might be at risk for developing or have already developed an addiction to exercise. The more TRUE answers you circled, the greater your risk of having an exercise addiction. You are probably experiencing issues in your life due to working out and exercising.

My Exercise Story TOTAL = _____

This assessment measures the impact of exercise habits on your health and life.

The HIGHER your score on the My Exercise Story Assessment
the more of an issue you have due to exercise addiction.

Not for Fun

People who use exercise to cope with stress, emotions, and unwanted thoughts often find exercise is no longer fun. It can lose its element of fun and play. It no longer serves a purpose. Exercise becomes a chore or something they MUST do. It is a job, an escape, and a duty.

In each of the hexagons below, write six words that describe the word exercise to you.

Words to Describe Exercise

© 2023 WHOLE PERSON ASSOCIATES, 101 WEST 2ND STREET, SUITE 203, DULUTH MN 55802 • 800-247-6789 • WHOLEPERSON.COM

My Exercise Addiction

People find many different ways to exercise and work out.

Following is a list of SOME of the ways people exercise.
Check off the ones that you do and write how often and why you like that form of exercise.

☐ Aerobic exercise _____

☐ Bicycle _____

☐ Bodyweight exercise _____

☐ Dance _____

☐ Fitness classes _____

☐ Golf _____

☐ Gymnastics _____

☐ Hike _____

☐ Jog _____

☐ Jump rope _____

☐ Kayak _____

☐ Marathon training _____

☐ Martial arts _____

☐ Push-ups _____

☐ Rock climbing _____

☐ Rollerblade or Skateboard _____

☐ Run _____

☐ Sport _____

☐ Swim/Dive _____

☐ Walk _____

☐ Weight Lift _____

☐ Workout video games _____

☐ Workout videos _____

☐ Zumba _____

What is your preferred method of exercise?_____

My SAFE Weekly Exercise Regimen (Part 1)

Regimen: a regulated course, as of diet, exercise, or manner of living, intended to preserve or restore health or attain some result.

Often, people who enjoy exercising set their workouts with a specific weekly regimen to which they intend to adhere. What is your basic regimen? Do you stick with it, not do it as much as you planned, or overdo it?

Every day, for one week, complete this chart.

Days of the Week	Activity	Amount of Time Planned No More than 1 Hour!	Hours Over (+) or Under (-) Planned Time
Monday			+ _____ - _____
Tuesday			+ _____ - _____
Wednesday			+ _____ - _____
Thursday			+ _____ - _____
Friday			+ _____ - _____
Saturday			+ _____ - _____
Sunday			+ _____ - _____

Hours under for the week _____ Hours over for the week _____

© 2023 WHOLE PERSON ASSOCIATES, 101 WEST 2ND STREET, SUITE 203, DULUTH MN 55802 • 800-247-6789 • WHOLEPERSON.COM

My SAFE Weekly Exercise Regimen (Part 2)

Many people addicted to exercise go above their intended workout regimen because of triggers in their environment. These triggers could include people (my partner makes me sad when he talks about money), stressors (I had a tight deadline at work and was utterly stressed), and situations that arise (my dog died). You can also reward yourself with positive affirmations when you have achieved a goal.

Using Part 1 of My SAFE Weekly Exercise Regimen, take the times you listed and write about them. What were the triggers, and how did you cope? BE HONEST!

Days of the Week	Triggers	How I Coped
Monday		
Tuesday		
Wednesday		
Thursday		
Friday		
Saturday		
Sunday		

What could you have handled differently? _____

_____

My PERFECT Weekly Exercise Regimen

You must set a specific weekly exercise regimen and stick to it. This regimen should be safe, healthy, and free of additional workouts or exercise hours.

Below, identify what you believe to be the perfect weekly exercise regimen. If there are days you do not plan to exercise, mark a zero in the Exercise Activities column.

Complete this chart every single day for a week.

Days of the Week	Exercise Activities	Start Time	Stop Time
Monday			
Tuesday			
Wednesday			
Thursday			
Friday			
Saturday			
Sunday			

What can you do to ensure you stick to your perfect weekly exercise regimen?

_____

_____

© 2023 WHOLE PERSON ASSOCIATES, 101 WEST 2ND STREET, SUITE 203, DULUTH MN 55802 • 800-247-6789 • WHOLEPERSON.COM

Am I Being Smart When I Extend Workouts?

People addicted to exercise often experience consequences when they extend their workouts. (Examples: late for family dinner, late for work, didn't get to a kid's concert, etc.) Extending a workout often includes extras like exercising for an extra hour, taking extra reps on the bench press, or running home after a hard soccer practice.

Think about the last week. Describe those times when you extended your exercise workouts, explain why you felt the need to do so, and describe whether it affected anyone else.

Times I Extended a Workout	Why I Extended It	Who or What Did It Af-fect?
Example: *I ran an extra three miles.*	*I kept thinking that I was getting fat and needed to keep going.*	*My family waited for me for dinner, and it was cold.*

How can you make sure you are exercising in a healthy manner?

_____

_____

How can you be sure you are considerate of the people important to you?

_____

_____

Compulsive Exercise: Help or Hurt?

Compulsive exercise is characterized by a craving for physical training, resulting in uncontrollable excessive exercise behavior with harmful consequences, such as injuries and impaired social relations.

Many people compulsively exercise. They do it for a variety of different reasons. It is important to explore whether you exercise compulsively and how.

Below, identify the reasons that you compulsively exercise, how it hurts or helps you, and things you could substitute so that you would not need to exercise so much.

Reasons I Exercise	Type of Exercise	How It Hurts or Helps Me
Example: I feel the excitement or rush of adrenaline.	*Running*	☒ HELPS *I am in the flow and feeling great!* ☐ HURTS ____
Example: I feel the excitement or rush of adrenaline.	*Running*	☐ HELPS ____ ☒ HURTS *I have a hard time walking the next day.*
Feel the excitement or rush of adrenaline		☐ HELPS ____ ☐ HURTS ____
To get away from people		☐ HELPS ____ ☐ HURTS ____
Numb negative feelings		☐ HELPS ____ ☐ HURTS ____
Avoid thinking about my problems		☐ HELPS ____ ☐ HURTS ____
Stop my boredom		☐ HELPS ____ ☐ HURTS ____
Lose weight and look or feel better		☐ HELPS ____ ☐ HURTS ____
Reduce stress		☐ HELPS ____ ☐ HURTS ____
Work off calories		☐ HELPS ____ ☐ HURTS ____
Other		☐ HELPS ____ ☐ HURTS ____

© 2023 WHOLE PERSON ASSOCIATES, 101 WEST 2ND STREET, SUITE 203, DULUTH MN 55802 • 800-247-6789 • WHOLEPERSON.COM

Other Issues

Many people who have an exercise addiction are also dealing with other issues. For example, a person who exercises a lot might also be coping with substance abuse issues, domestic violence, mental health concerns, depression, eating disorders like anorexia nervosa or bulimia nervosa, body image issues, impulse control issues, partner problems, kid's issues, etc.

What issues are you dealing with in addition to excessive exercise? Write them in the circles below. In the space next to each one, describe what you are doing to cope with that issue.

My Other Issues

What is Healthy Exercise?

If you are compulsively exercising and hurting your body, you must reflect on what constitutes healthy exercise. How important is it to stick to a specific workout regimen, refuse to do anything extra, and know when to stop?

Discuss what constitutes healthy exercise for you on the lines below. Use a separate section for your conceptions of what that would be for you. Add an extra page if necessary.

To me, healthy exercise means ...

Example: Walking a mile a day, engaging in one of the martial arts, trying yoga.

_____

_____

_____

_____

_____

_____

_____

_____

To me, unhealthy exercise means ...

Example: Working out at the gym until I am in pain.

_____

_____

_____

_____

_____

_____

_____

_____

© 2023 WHOLE PERSON ASSOCIATES, 101 WEST 2ND STREET, SUITE 203, DULUTH MN 55802 • 800-247-6789 • WHOLEPERSON.COM

Recommended Daily Exercise Guidelines

Some people believe that the more they exercise, the better it is for their bodies. Unfortunately, this is not always the case. *The American College of Sports Medicine* guidelines presents a way to develop a healthy exercise plan and stick with it.

Explore each of the guidelines below. Write how you can stick to them, exceed them, or choose not to do that type of exercise.

Cardiorespiratory Exercise: Adults should get at least 150 minutes of moderate-intensity exercise per week. Exercise recommendations can be met through 30 to 60 minutes of moderate-intensity exercise five days per week or 20 to 60 minutes of vigorous-intensity exercise three days per week. One continuous session and multiple shorter sessions of at least 10 minutes are acceptable to accumulate the desired amount of daily routine.

_____

_____

Resistance Exercise: Adults should train each major muscle group two or three days each week using a variety of exercises and equipment. Very light or light intensity is best for older individuals or previously sedentary adults just starting to exercise. Two to four sets of each exercise, with anywhere between eight and 20 repetitions, will help adults improve strength and power.

_____

_____

Flexibility Exercise: Adults should do flexibility exercises at least two or three days each week to improve range of motion. Each stretch should be held for 10 to 30 seconds to the point of tightness or slight discomfort. Repeat each stretch two to four times, accumulating 60 seconds per stretch.

_____

_____

Neuromotor Exercise: Neuromotor exercise, also referred to as "functional fitness training," is recommended two or three days per week. Exercises should involve motor skills (balance, agility, coordination, and gait), muscle flexibility training, and multifaceted activities (yoga) to improve physical function and prevent falls in older adults. Between 20 and 30 minutes of exercise per day is appropriate for neuromotor exercise.

_____

_____

Perhaps you can add the above types of exercise and do less of other varieties.

My Exercise and Workout History

Most people follow specific patterns in their life workouts and exercise sessions. This page will help you explore your history related to exercise.

Complete each sentence starter by writing about your own experiences with exercising. What patterns do you notice?

I first started working out when I was _____ years old.

The person who aroused my interest in working out was (USE NAME CODE) _____

This person exercised this way_____

_____

The first time I worked out with someone was with (USE NAME CODE)_____

The exercises I did with this person were _____

_____

(Circle) I liked / didn't like / loved / hated doing the exercise this person did. Why? _____

_____

(Circle) Over my childhood years, I have always / sometimes / never exercised. Explain. _____

_____

I started exercising seriously (when?) _____

_____

In recent years I have exercised (circle) regularly / not enough / too much / sometimes / once in a while. Explain. _____

(Circle) Now, I work out constantly / here and there / way too much / hardly ever / only when I am unhappy / when I am happy/other. Explain. _____

Now, I work out this often because _____

_____

I tend to work out after talking with (NAME CODE) _____

Why?_____

_____

Exercise has positively affected my life by_____

_____

Exercise has negatively affected my life by _____

_____

© 2023 WHOLE PERSON ASSOCIATES, 101 WEST 2ND STREET, SUITE 203, DULUTH MN 55802 • 800-247-6789 • WHOLEPERSON.COM

Time to Reflect

Reflection: to give serious thought or consideration.

Following are some questions for your reflection. Provide your responses in the spaces that follow each reflective question.

How do you know when you have exercised too much or reached your limits?

_____

_____

How can you keep yourself from exercising more when you reach your limits?

_____

_____

If you feel you have done too much, what do you do to ensure that you recover properly?

_____

_____

How do you know when you are ready to resume your normal exercise routine after doing too much?

_____

_____

When you have been ill, injured, or do not feel like exercising, do you continue to exercise? If so, why? If not, why?

_____

_____

How could you modify your training to accommodate an illness or injury?

_____

_____

If you don't like something change it; if you can't change it,
change the way you think about it.
~ Mary Engelbreit

When I Overexercise

It's very healthy for you to exercise and work out. However, it works against you and your body when you become obsessed with exercise and overdo it. Your body begins to break down and needs some rest.

Draw or doodle your responses.

What Do You Look Like After You Overdo Your Exercise?	What Type of Less Intense Form of Workout Can You Do?
What Type of Activity Do You Choose As Your Exercise Regimen?	**When You Tend to Overdo, What Is a Less-Intense Workout You Could Be Doing?**

© 2023 WHOLE PERSON ASSOCIATES, 101 WEST 2ND STREET, SUITE 203, DULUTH MN 55802 • 800-247-6789 • WHOLEPERSON.COM

Costs of Excessive Exercise

How is your excessive exercise negatively affecting your life?

On the line under each of the ways exercising affects you; place an X on the continuum based on how you see yourself. On the dotted line below, write why you rated yourself that way. BE HONEST!

I am so obsessed I do not want to do anything else but exercise.

0 (Not Like Me)   5 (Somewhat Like Me)   10 (Much Like Me)

I get cranky, disagreeable, and angry when I am not exercising.

0 (Not Like Me)   5 (Somewhat Like Me)   10 (Much Like Me)

I feel like I have no excitement or pleasure in my life other than exercising.

0 (Not Like Me)   5 (Somewhat Like Me)   10 (Much Like Me)

My work has suffered because of my overexercising.

0 (Not Like Me)   5 (Somewhat Like Me)   10 (Much Like Me)

I don't believe my health problems are from too much exercise.

0 (Not Like Me)   5 (Somewhat Like Me)   10 (Much Like Me)

My body hurts most of the time.

0 (Not Like Me)   5 (Somewhat Like Me)   10 (Much Like Me)

HIGHER SCORES (Much Like Me) on many of the statements indicate that you probably have an exercise addiction.

MEDIUM SCORES (Somewhat Like Me) other than getting a zero indicate a possible exercise addiction problem.

LOWER SCORES (Not Like Me) suggest that you are not experiencing many signs of an exercise problem.

Case Study

GFW works out twice a day, seven days a week. He usually spends 10 hours at the boxing gym each week. When he is not at the gym, he goes on long daily runs and even squeezes in an hour of yoga, Pilates, or tai chi every morning. He even exercises on holidays. He never rests. He has limited relationships.

Do you think that GFW has a problem or not?

_____

_____

_____

What do you think about his workout regimen?

_____

_____

Is this like your exercise program? Is it similar? Does it differ? In what ways?

_____

_____

_____

How could GFW begin to slow down overexercising?

_____

_____

_____

How do you think GFW's exercise program affects his life and relationships?

_____

_____

_____

How does your exercise program affect your life and relationships?

_____

_____

_____

© 2023 WHOLE PERSON ASSOCIATES, 101 WEST 2ND STREET, SUITE 203, DULUTH MN 55802 • 800-247-6789 • WHOLEPERSON.COM

Quotes about Overexercising

*On the lines that follow each of the quotes, describe what the
quote means to you and how it applies to YOUR life.*

There are three methods to gaining wisdom. The first is reflection, which is the
highest. The second is limitation, which is the easiest.
The third is experience, which is the bitterest.
~ Confucius

_____

_____

I try and work out as much as I can because when you exercise, it releases endorphins
and makes you feel really good. I also make sure I schedule time with my friends,
family, and loved ones because I realize that, as well as your physical well-being, you
have to look out for your mental well-being, too.
~ Philomena Kwao

_____

_____

The difference is that a compulsive exerciser works out not to
feel good but to avoid feeling bad.
~ Carolyn Plateau

_____

_____

I exercised to avoid feeling anxious or tense–
because I knew how bad I'd feel if I didn't.
~ Mary E. Pritchard

_____

_____

Which quote especially speaks to you about your overexercising? Why?

_____

_____

_____

_____

© 2023 WHOLE PERSON ASSOCIATES, 101 WEST 2ND STREET, SUITE 203, DULUTH MN 55802 • 800-247-6789 • WHOLEPERSON.COM

Exercise

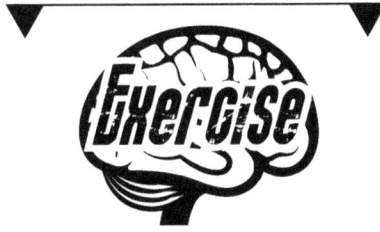

Coping with Compulsion

Name _____

Date _____

© 2023 WHOLE PERSON ASSOCIATES, 101 WEST 2ND STREET, SUITE 203, DULUTH MN 55802 • 800-247-6789 • WHOLEPERSON.COM

Coping with Compulsion Assessment
Introduction and Directions

Compulsion: Any action taken because of obsessive thoughts.

Many people work out excessively because they cannot cope with stress, anxiety, and compulsive thinking. The *Coping with Compulsion Assessment* was designed to help you explore why you may use exercise to cope with life problems and challenges.

This assessment contains 15 statements that measure the three ways people use excessive exercise as a crutch to cope instead of relying on healthier coping tools and techniques.

Read each of the statements and decide whether it describes you. If it is TRUE, circle the number next to that item under the TRUE column. If it is FALSE, circle the number next to that item under the FALSE column.

In the following example, the circled 2 indicates that the person completing this assessment believes that the statement is true for them:

STRESS SCALE	TRUE	FALSE
When it comes to exercising ...		
I use it to deal with stress	(2)	1
I like that it takes me away from my problems	(2)	1

This is not a test. Since there are no right or wrong answers, do not spend too much time thinking about them. Be sure to respond to every statement.

BE HONEST!

If you choose, no one else needs to see the results.

(Turn to the next page and begin.)

© 2023 WHOLE PERSON ASSOCIATES, 101 WEST 2ND STREET, SUITE 203, DULUTH MN 55802 • 800-247-6789 • WHOLEPERSON.COM

Coping with Compulsion Assessment

Name _____ Date _____

This will only be accurate if you respond honestly. No one else needs to see this if you choose.

STRESS SCALE
	TRUE	FALSE

When it comes to exercising ...

I use it to deal with stress 2 1

I like that it takes me away from my problems. 2 1

I exercise instead of dealing with relationship issues 2 1

I feel more confident and in control when I am working out 2 1

I use it to reduce anxiety 2 1

Stress Scale TOTAL = _____

MY THOUGHTS SCALE
	TRUE	FALSE

When it comes to exercising ...

I have negative thoughts about myself. 2 1

I have a constant stream of thoughts going on in my head about exercising. .2 1

I believe that I am not successful unless I overtrain. 2 1

I have thoughts that keep pushing me to train more and more 2 1

I believe I am obese and out of shape, even though I don't want to be 2 1

My Thoughts Scale TOTAL = _____

CONTROL SCALE
	TRUE	FALSE

When it comes to exercising ...

I cannot control the amount of time I exercise 2 1

I feel like I never reach my full exercise potential 2 1

I am not able to stop myself from exercising. 2 1

I feel helpless to change my actions despite the physical consequences. . . .2 1

I try to control what happens in my life by exercising. 2 1

Control Scale TOTAL = _____

Go to the next page for scoring assessment results, profile interpretation, and individual description.

© 2023 WHOLE PERSON ASSOCIATES, 101 WEST 2ND STREET, SUITE 203, DULUTH MN 55802 • 800-247-6789 • WHOLEPERSON.COM

Coping With Compulsion Assessment

Descriptions and Profile Interpretation

The assessment you just completed examines ways people use exercise to cope with life.

Add the scores you circled on the previous page and put that number in the TOTAL space.
Transfer that number below. Then place each number on the continuum line of the matching scale:

Assessment Profile Interpretation

Stress Scale – This scale measures how much you use exercise to cope with stressors.

_____
5 = Low   8 = Moderate   10 = High

My Thoughts Scale – This scale measures how much you use exercise to cope with negative thinking.

_____
5 = Low   8 = Moderate   10 = High

Control Scale – This scale measures how much you exercise because you cannot control your impulses.

_____
5 = Low   8 = Moderate   10 = High

The higher your score on any of the scales, the more you use working out and excessive exercise to cope with life, and the greater your risk of experiencing the negative effects of exercise addiction.

By circling even ONE Moderate or High answer, you risk experiencing the negative effects of excessive exercise on your personal and professional life.

What surprises you the most about your scores?

_____

_____

_____

What surprises you the least about your scores?

_____

_____

_____

My Awareness

It is vital to cultivate an awareness of your thoughts and behaviors surrounding exercise. You can begin by identifying thoughts about your problematic relationship to exercise. Notice the thoughts that you have regarding exercise. Do you tell yourself, "A workout does not count unless I sweat?" Maybe you think, "I can eat as much as I want as long as I exercise more than usual."

Below, list your unhealthy thoughts tied to exercising. Then identify healthier thoughts.

My Unhealthy Thoughts Tied to Exercising	Healthier Thoughts Tied to Exercising
Example: I must work out twice a day or become fat and lazy!	*Working out once a day is enough, and it will give me more time with my family.*

Many people in this world are still so identified with every thought that arises in their head. There is not the slightest space of awareness there.
~ Eckhart Tolle

 © 2023 WHOLE PERSON ASSOCIATES, 101 WEST 2ND STREET, SUITE 203, DULUTH MN 55802 • 800-247-6789 • WHOLEPERSON.COM

In Control of Your Impulses?

Impulse: a sudden spontaneous inclination or incitement to some usually unpremeditated action

Many people who overexercise do it because they cannot control their impulses. They experience an emotion, feel stressed, cannot control it, and impulsively turn to what they know – exercise – to solve their problem!

Respond to the table below about impulses and exercise.

Who or What Prompted One of My Impulses? USE NAME CODES.	The Impulse	The Exercise
Example: HGA refused to go on a date with me. I was so sad!	*I felt the immediate need to exercise and try to forget about it.*	*I ran three miles, rested, and ran another three miles.*

Managing a Compulsion

Managing: handling or directing with a degree of skill
Compulsion: an irresistible persistent impulse

Usually, those who overexercise have persistent impulses. Become aware of your compulsions. Compulsion control will help manage the wave of urges that prompt addictive behavior. You may experience unwanted thoughts triggering anxiety, distress, and fears. The compulsion to exercise is an attempt to neutralize your fears or make obsessive thoughts disappear. When having these unwanted thoughts that you try to squelch through exercise, the following steps are helpful:

- Put off the craving for as long as you can. *(Count to 20, take deep breaths, etc.)*
- Remove yourself from the situation if possible. *(Walk away, listen to music, etc.)*
- Avoid any triggers that prompt you to engage in exercise. *(Avoid talking with a friend who always wants to exercise; avoid driving by the gym, etc.)*
- Do something else you enjoy. *(Read a good book, go to a movie, play cards with friends, etc.)*

Think of how you can deal with compulsive urges:

Name a situation in which you had an urge to exercise._____

_____

How could you have put off the craving?_____

_____

How could you have removed yourself from the situation? _____

_____

How could you have avoided triggers to exercise? _____

_____

Name three other things you enjoy that you could have done instead of exercise or people you could have joined:

1 _____.

2. _____

3. _____

© 2023 WHOLE PERSON ASSOCIATES, 101 WEST 2ND STREET, SUITE 203, DULUTH MN 55802 • 800-247-6789 • WHOLEPERSON.COM

Thinking About Warning Signs

You might suspect (or know) that you have a problem with exercising. You probably overexercise, work out too many times per day, or exercise even when you are sick or hurt. It is important to know whether you are struggling with any other warning signs indicating that your relationship to exercise and working out is unhealthy.

Refer to the warning signs below and identify your unrealistic thoughts about the statement.

Example: Exercising despite illness or injury because...
- *No injury will keep me down!*
- *Only wimps allow an injury to keep them from working out!*
- *If I don't show up to exercise even though I am sick, it will show that I am weak.*

Explain if these thoughts are true about you. Why or why not?

I exercise despite illness or injury.

_____

_____

I feel anxious or guilty if my exercise routine is disrupted.

_____

_____

I would rather give up or avoid social events than give up exercise.

_____

_____

No matter how rigid my exercise routine is, I never feel it is too severe.

_____

_____

I do not feel I can take off even one day to rest from exercising.

_____

_____

Discuss your responses with someone you trust.

Healthy Coping Statements

Healthy coping statements will encourage you. They will help you manage distressing and challenging circumstances and will help deal with your compulsive reactions to your exercise urges.

Fill in the remaining boxes with your coping statements.

When I need to exercise no matter what, this too will pass.	Take some time to stop and breathe rather than exercise.	I am strong. I can resist the urge to overexercise.

© 2023 WHOLE PERSON ASSOCIATES, 101 WEST 2ND STREET, SUITE 203, DULUTH MN 55802 • 800-247-6789 • WHOLEPERSON.COM

Challenge Exercise Rules

Many people addicted to exercise have a long list of exercise rules they feel they MUST follow.

Identify your exercise rules, and then write some healthier rules you can follow.

My Exercise Rules	Healthier Rules
Example: I cannot take any days off, or my exercise program will fail.	*I can exercise three days a week and take the other days to spend with my friends and family.*
Example: I must exercise twice every day, or I will get fat.	*I can control my being fat by exercising four days a week and eating less junk food!*
Example: I cannot take any days off each week, or I will begin taking off even more days.	*I will write the days I need to exercise on a calendar and put a checkmark after exercising.*

Tips for Developing New Exercise Rules
- Gradually work on challenging your old rules in small and manageable steps. The above method for challenging these thoughts will help.
- Start by taking one rest day a week or trying a gentle yoga class instead of running.
- Shave off 10 minutes of your daily exercise routine.
- Even though you feel bad about missing exercise time, this feeling will pass. Do not give in to it.
- Find some forms of movement that you can enjoy which will provide variety, flexibility, and healthy balance.

Processing Your Emotions

Many people who work out regularly use exercise to deal with the emotions they are experiencing. Often, rather than deal with their negative emotions in a healthy manner, they overexercise. They usually believe using exercise to relieve powerful emotions makes sense. It becomes a problem when this is the primary way people cope with emotions. People need to have a variety of ways to process and distract with coping strategies.

Below, write about the situations that trigger your powerful, negative emotions.

Situations That Trigger My Powerful, Negative Emotions	Ways I Cope with the Emotions Using Exercise	The Effect This Is Having on Me and Others in My Life
Example: I got into an argument with my girlfriend, felt angry and hopeless, and stormed out of the room.	*I isolated myself in the basement and did a bunch of reps to push the anger down.*	*This cycle repeats itself because I'm ashamed to tell her that I'm feeling lost in life.*

Let's explore a processing format you can use to deal with your emotions.
The next time you experience powerful, negative emotions, try this process to relieve them:

Step 1: Take Time to Pause
Stop yourself and block the behavior instead of compulsively acting on feelings immediately. You can try counting to 50 or reciting the alphabet backward.

Step 2: Acknowledge Your Feelings
Name the feelings you are experiencing. If you are angry, try to determine if you are frustrated, furious, steamed, or all of the above.

Step 3: Think about Your Thinking
This may sound strange, but it works. Think about why you are experiencing the emotion. Do you feel insulted by what was said or done? Are your feelings hurt? Or is it that your thinking makes you angry? Whatever it is that you are feeling, it's okay! Now that you have taken a few moments to figure out exactly what you are feeling, think about how you can make yourself feel better.

Step 4: Take Action
Take action to help yourself deal with negative thoughts. This might include being mindful and noticing your surroundings, changing your thinking to be more positive, or finding a new distraction.

 © 2023 WHOLE PERSON ASSOCIATES, 101 WEST 2ND STREET, SUITE 203, DULUTH MN 55802 • 800-247-6789 • WHOLEPERSON.COM

Distracting Yourself

Many people can't stop thinking about exercising. They get up in the morning thinking about their workout regimen, exercise during the day, and go to sleep at night thinking about how they will exercise the next day or what they should have done today. If your thinking becomes obsessive and your focus on working out begins to get in the way of doing regular healthy tasks, it becomes a troubling obsession.

Rather than compulsively turning to exercise, you may want to try to feel a sense of calm with mindful activities such as meditation, artwork, journaling, having a massage, or talking to a friend. What are some ways you could distract yourself when you feel powerful emotions?

In each of the four blocks below, write about, draw, or doodle a way you can distract yourself with a mindful activity.

1.	2.
3.	4.

When there are thoughts, it is distraction: when there are no thoughts, it is meditation.
~ Ramana Maharshi

What's Bothering You?

Many people who are addicted to exercise attempt to numb out through exercise. They do not want to deal with stress, emotions, anxiety, frustration, etc. In these cases, working out becomes a temporary Band-Aid to cope with or fix the problem for a permanent solution.

In the circles below, identify what is bothering you. If you can do this, you can process negative thoughts in a healthy manner so that you do not have to rely on excessive exercise. In the space next to each circle, identify a solution to the problem.

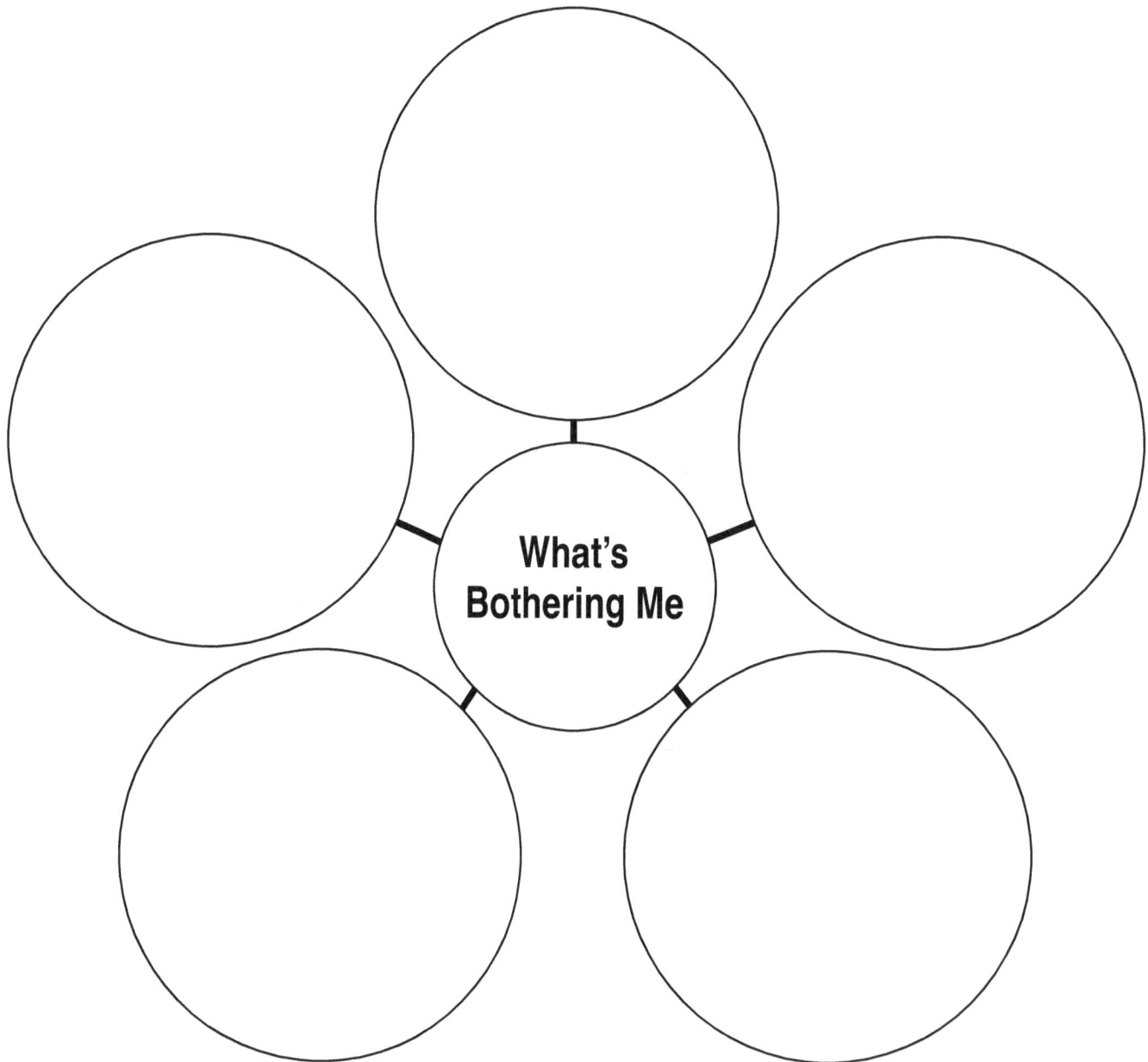

What's Bothering Me

Once you write it, you can deal with it.
~ Niki Tilicki

© 2023 WHOLE PERSON ASSOCIATES, 101 WEST 2ND STREET, SUITE 203, DULUTH MN 55802 • 800-247-6789 • WHOLEPERSON.COM

Dealing with Stress

Everyone experiences stress. We are meant to feel stress. We are meant to react to it. It keeps us alert. However, stress becomes a problem when it persists. One of the most critical life skills is dealing with stress effectively. Rather than overexercising, you might journal how you feel, scream into a pillow, share your feelings with someone you trust, cry, etc.

Below, identify some healthy ways to deal with your stress such as working out in a healthy, reasonable way.

Stress I Experienced (USE NAME CODES)	How I Dealt With it through Overexercise	How I Could Have Coped in a Better Way
Example: MSM was in the hospital and was very ill.	I visited him in the hospital every day and then exercised for hours, so I would be able to fall asleep.	I love to do artwork. I could have gone home and made some cards to give him every day.

It's not stress that kills us, it is our reaction to it.
~ Hans Selye

What does the above quote mean to you?

_____

_____

What are four ways you can react to stress without exercising?

1. _____

2. _____

3. _____

4. _____

Obsessive Thinking

When people overexercise, it is often due to obsessive thinking about their fitness, exercise regimen, or appearance. Obsessive thinking triggers them to exercise compulsively.

With each of the obsessive thoughts below, write a healthier, less obsessive thought.

Example
Obsessive Thought: I strain a quad in spin class. I think, "I need to exercise every day," so I ice it, heat it, wrap it, take a few painkillers, and then start my exercise regimen again the next day.
Healthy Thought: I strain a quad in spin class. I think, "I don't need to exercise every day. It's okay to take some time off. Taking time off is not a sign of weakness. It could help me heal."

Obsessive Thought: I eat a big meal and top it off with dessert at a friend's birthday dinner. I think, "That is the last time I am eating out with friends!"

Healthy Thought: _____

_____

Obsessive Thought: I exercised so much that I slept in and missed an important business meeting in the morning. I think, "I will not schedule any more meetings in the morning."

Healthy Thought: _____

_____

Obsessive Thought: I have no time to cook, so I go to a take-out restaurant. I buy some food and take it home. When I get home, I think, "I'll never be able to exercise enough to work off all the calories and carbs." I throw the food away.

Healthy Thought: _____

_____

Write about one of your past experiences when you reacted in an obsessive way regarding exercise.

_____

_____

What could have been a healthy thought in this situation? _____

_____

© 2023 WHOLE PERSON ASSOCIATES, 101 WEST 2ND STREET, SUITE 203, DULUTH MN 55802 • 800-247-6789 • WHOLEPERSON.COM

Appreciation

Excessive workouts decrease your appreciation for people and things in your life.

Below, identify the things you appreciate in your life.

Things In My Life I Appreciate	Why I Appreciate Them	Ways I Can Be Involved
Example: Woodworking.	*I love creating things with my hands.*	*I can work on that cabinet I wanted to make instead of overexercising.*

Below, identify the people you appreciate in your life.

People In My Life I Appreciate	Why I Appreciate Them	How I Can Be More Involved
Example: My children.	*They make me laugh and keep me feeling young.*	*I can spend more time with them and less time at the gym.*

Stress Quote

Read the following quotation and respond to the questions below.

If it's stress of things that we cannot control, what you have to do is you mitigate that stress as much as possible. You've planned, you've trained, you've done everything you can in your power to mitigate the stress that's facing you. And then after that, there's nothing you can do.
So, you have to let that one go.
~ Jocko Willink

What does this quote mean to you?

_____
_____
_____

How does exercise help alleviate stress?

_____
_____
_____

What about your life is out of your control?

_____
_____
_____

How do you alleviate stress other than exercising?

_____
_____
_____

How can you plan better to alleviate your stress?

_____
_____
_____

How can you let go of things you cannot control?

_____
_____
_____

© 2023 WHOLE PERSON ASSOCIATES, 101 WEST 2ND STREET, SUITE 203, DULUTH MN 55802 • 800-247-6789 • WHOLEPERSON.COM

Mindfulness

At times, we all fall into habits of mind and body, attention and inattention, which result in not being present in our lives. People who overexercise often get caught up in their workout regimen and fail to remain aware of their surroundings. One way to stop the compulsive reaction to stress or challenging emotions is to be mindful.

An important antidote to the tendency to tune out and go on automatic pilot is to practice mindfulness.

Think about the last time you were stressed. What was the situation?

_____

Notice the stress in your body. When you encounter stress or adversity in your life, shape it rather than being a bystander. Shaping your experiences means learning to pay attention to what is occurring in your body. In your situation, what could you have noticed about how you were feeling stress?

_____

_____

Try to relax. Take a few deep breaths. This relaxed feeling helps you to be more present and mindful. In your situation, how could you have relaxed more?

_____

_____

_____

Be mindful. Stay in the present by noticing noises, sights, and smells. Take deep breaths. In your situation, what did you notice?

_____

_____

_____

Practice staying present. By not turning away from stress in your life, you will learn to remain open to the possibilities in each situation. You will not rush to exercise to relieve your stress. In your situation, how could you have stayed present with the stress?

_____

_____

_____

It is possible that the stress would have passed without you having to work out!

Mood-Altering Effects

Overexercising, like any other compulsion, is maintained for its mood-altering effects. There are healthy mood-improving effects of exercise until it becomes an obsession.

In the hexagrams below, identify some of the other types of activities that bring you joy and alter your mood positively.

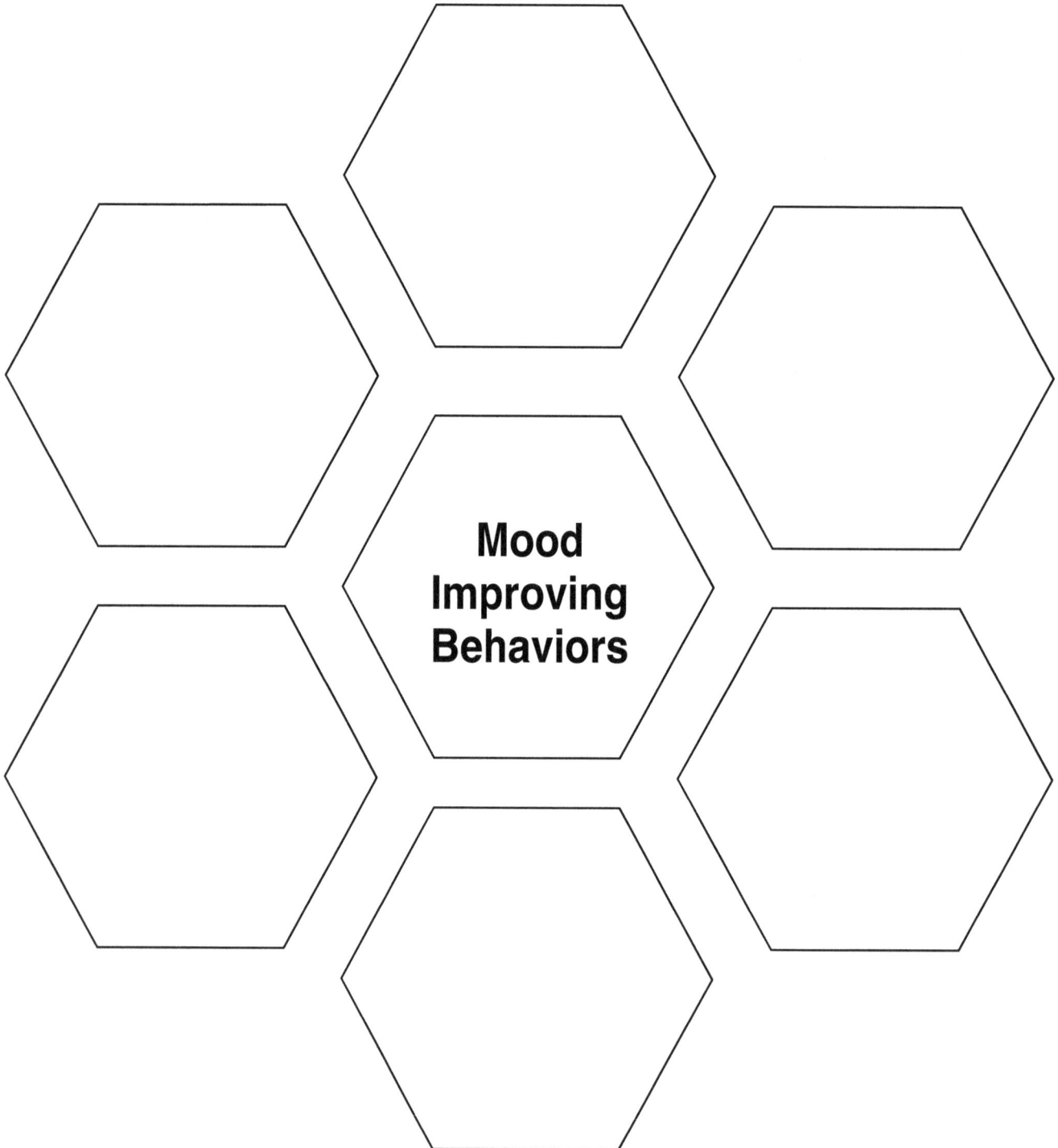

Mood Improving Behaviors

© 2023 WHOLE PERSON ASSOCIATES, 101 WEST 2ND STREET, SUITE 203, DULUTH MN 55802 • 800-247-6789 • WHOLEPERSON.COM

Quotes About Coping

On the lines that follow each of the quotes, describe what the quote means to you and how it applies to your compulsions to exercise .

When I started training, I just started running every day, which you shouldn't do. I learned that lesson the hard way by getting a stress fracture.
~ Sophia Bush

_____

_____

In times of great stress or adversity, it's always best to keep busy, to plow your anger and your energy into something positive.
~ Lee Iacocca

_____

_____

Sometimes you have compulsions that you can't control coming from the subconscious... they are the dictator inside ourselves.
~ Denis Villeneuve

_____

_____

I'm not very good at talking about my emotions.
~ Caroline Flack

_____

_____

Which quote especially speaks to you about overexercising? Why?

_____

_____

_____

_____

_____

_____

© 2023 WHOLE PERSON ASSOCIATES, 101 WEST 2ND STREET, SUITE 203, DULUTH MN 55802 • 800-247-6789 • WHOLEPERSON.COM

Exercise

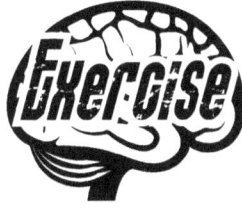

Problem Behavior

Name _____

Date _____

© 2023 WHOLE PERSON ASSOCIATES, 101 WEST 2ND STREET, SUITE 203, DULUTH MN 55802 • 800-247-6789 • WHOLEPERSON.COM

© 2023 WHOLE PERSON ASSOCIATES, 101 WEST 2ND STREET, SUITE 203, DULUTH MN 55802 • 800-247-6789 • WHOLEPERSON.COM

Problem Behavior Assessment
Introduction and Directions

Exercise is good for everyone. It enhances the quality of life by improving moods, boosting energy, promoting better sleep, controlling weight, and combating some health conditions. However, when someone is addicted to exercise, it no longer improves the quality of life. On the contrary, overexercising causes problems in a person's life in both physical and psychological ways.

The Problem Behavior Assessment contains 20 statements related to problem behaviors experienced by people with exercise addiction.

Read each of the statements and decide if it describes you. If it describes you, circle the YES column next to that item. If it does not describe you, circle the NO column next to that item.

In the following example, the circled YES indicates that the statement describes the person completing this assessment:

When it comes to my overexercising behavior ...

I have lost many of my non-workout friends. . . . . (YES) . . . . NO

I am often anxious, irritable, or angry . . . . (YES) . . . . NO

This is not a test. Since there are no right or wrong answers, do not spend too much time thinking about them. Be sure to respond to every statement.

BE HONEST!

If you choose, no one else needs to see the results.

(Turn to the next page and begin.)

Problem Behavior Assessment

Name _____ Date _____

This will only be accurate if you respond honestly. No one else needs to see this if you choose.

When it comes to my overexercising behavior ...

I have lost many of my non-workout friends.............................YES..........NO

I am often anxious, irritable, or angry ....YES..........NO

I have many medical problems..YES..........NO

I have had a significant decrease in motivation or enjoyment.............YES..........NO

I have had a drop in my workout performance ....YES..........NO

I need longer periods of rest ....YES..........NO

I become depressed when I cannot exercise...............................YES..........NO

I forget to drink a lot of water or eat food before I work out ....YES..........NO

I am unable to perform at the same level ....YES..........NO

I have sore muscles a lot of the time.......................................YES..........NO

I get more colds...YES..........NO

I am losing weight and need to remember to eat healthy foods ....YES..........NO

I am not motivated to do anything else but exercise ....YES..........NO

I am having family issues...YES..........NO

I have impulse-control problems...YES..........NO

I have trouble sleeping...YES..........NO

I have sudden mood changes...YES..........NO

I feel fatigued a lot of the time..YES..........NO

I no longer perform basic daily tasks ....YES..........NO

I am not interested in sex anymore...YES..........NO

TOTAL "YES" Answers = _____

Go to the next page for scoring assessment results,
profile interpretation, and individual description.

  © 2023 WHOLE PERSON ASSOCIATES, 101 WEST 2ND STREET, SUITE 203, DULUTH MN 55802 • 800-247-6789 • WHOLEPERSON.COM

Problem Behavior Assessment

Descriptions and Profile Interpretation

The assessment you just completed is designed to measure the impact of excessive exercise on your career, health, relationships, and life overall.

Count the number of YES answers you circled on the Problem Behavior Assessment. Put that total on the line marked TOTAL at the end of the section on the assessment. Transfer your total to this space below:

Problem Behavior TOTAL = _____

Assessment Profile Interpretation

By circling even ONE Yes answer, you risk developing or having an exercise addiction. The more Yes answers you circled, the greater your chance of experiencing an extensive problem with your exercising behavior.

The HIGHER your score on the Problem Behavior Assessment, the more issues you have due to your exercise behavior. Place an X on the line below for your score

.

This assessment measures the impact of overexercising on your life.

0 = Low	10 = Moderate	20 = High

What is your reaction to your score?

_____

_____

_____

_____

_____

Social Commitments

People addicted to exercise often want to do nothing but work out. They end up missing many social events, or they break a promise to meet somewhere and leave the person waiting, all because of their exercise routine. These missed social commitments can cause serious problems with partners, children, co-workers, family, friends, etc., especially when they happen more than once.

Below, identify the times you missed any type of social commitment due to exercising.

Missed Social Commitments (USE NAME CODES)	What It Had to Do with My Exercising	How It Affected My Life and Other's Lives
CHD's 16th birthday party.	I was working out at the gym and didn't look at the time.	She was devastated, and I am told she cried throughout her party and kept looking out the window!

The one thing I regret is missing the time with
my older children when they were young.
~ Kris Kristofferson

© 2023 WHOLE PERSON ASSOCIATES, 101 WEST 2ND STREET, SUITE 203, DULUTH MN 55802 • 800-247-6789 • WHOLEPERSON.COM

Loss of Interest

One of the symptoms of people who overexercise is losing interest in their hobbies, activities, or even friends and family. The chances are that these people are not actually bored with their hobbies, activities, friends, or family because they want to use that time to exercise.

Think about your hobbies (example, artwork), activities (example, bowling in a league), close family (example, going to a movie with them once a week), or friends (example, having coffee with your best friend every other week) that you have given up on because of your obsession with exercise.

Draw, doodle, or write about your "loss of interest" in one of each of these categories:

A Hobby	An Activity

Family	A Friend

Preferences

Often, people like to exercise so much that they slowly start exercising more and more and soon are overexercising. When exercising becomes more satisfying, and you prefer it more than other pleasant activities such as going out with friends and family, eating at a special restaurant, or celebrating special occasions, it can become a big problem.

Identify some ways you prefer exercise over other pleasant activities in life.
No one else needs to see this paper. It's for your awareness.
BE HONEST!

Example: I prefer exercising and working out to going to my job, where I sit all day long for eight hours! Why is this? I probably could get up from time to time, but then I won't get as much done, and I'm not particularly eager to gossip with everyone when they walk around.

I prefer exercising and working out to _____

Why is this? _____

_____

I prefer exercising and working out to _____

Why is this? _____

_____

I prefer exercising and working out to _____

Why is this? _____

_____

I prefer exercising and working out to _____

Why is this? _____

_____

I prefer exercising and working out to _____

Why is this? _____

_____

© 2023 WHOLE PERSON ASSOCIATES, 101 WEST 2ND STREET, SUITE 203, DULUTH MN 55802 • 800-247-6789 • WHOLEPERSON.COM

Energy Imbalance

Energy Imbalance: The difference between the amount of energy consumed and the amount of energy expended.

Overexercising can cause an energy imbalance. Over an extended period, people with an energy deficit can have many issues: sadness, burnout, loneliness, guilt, shame, etc.

Complete each sentence starter below by listing the things you do not have the energy for and how not doing them hurts you and the significant others in your life.

For Example:
I don't have the energy to go out with friends. I am lonely but can't stop working out.

I don't have the energy to... _____

_____

_____

I don't have the energy to... _____

_____

_____

I don't have the energy to... _____

_____

_____

I don't have the energy to... _____

_____

_____

I don't have the energy to... _____

_____

_____

I don't have the energy to... _____

_____

_____

In addition to working out less, here are other ways to increase your energy:
- Balance work and rest.
- Try to streamline your list of "must-do" exercise regimens.
- Set your priorities in terms of the most important non-exercise tasks.
- Replace addictive thoughts (I must, I should, If I don't) with more positive thoughts based on a more balanced lifestyle.
- Get as much sleep as you possibly can. Avoid working out too close to your bedtime.
- Learn to control stress in ways other than exercising. Relaxation through meditation, yoga, and tai chi are also effective tools for reducing stress.

A Financial Drain?

Does exercise create a financial drain for you and your family? Exercise equipment, gym membership, and workout clothes can be expensive and are often used as motivators by those who are exercising.

Identify some of the exercise-related expenses that you have incurred and the outcomes.

My Exercise Purchases in the Last 12 Months.	How I Use the Purchases as an Excuse to Exercise	Is It Depriving Me or Anyone in My Family Because of the Expense? Explain.
Example: I paid a tremendous amount of money for my equipment to be able to exercise at home.	*I spent all that money and need to get my money's worth!*	*I charged the equipment, and I am paying it monthly. We are barely squeaking by because of the payments.*

To own up to one's lack of courage and shortcoming without excuses is courage.
~ Jesse Lee Peterson

© 2023 WHOLE PERSON ASSOCIATES, 101 WEST 2ND STREET, SUITE 203, DULUTH MN 55802 • 800-247-6789 • WHOLEPERSON.COM

Trouble Paying the Bills?

Many people who struggle with excessive exercise end up missing work due to exercising *(recovering from exercise sessions, thinking about exercise sessions, or preparing to exercise)*. They miss so much work that they can no longer successfully pay the bills, or they are spending more than they can afford. This is an indicator that a problem exists!

Below, identify the times you missed work due to exercising and the result.

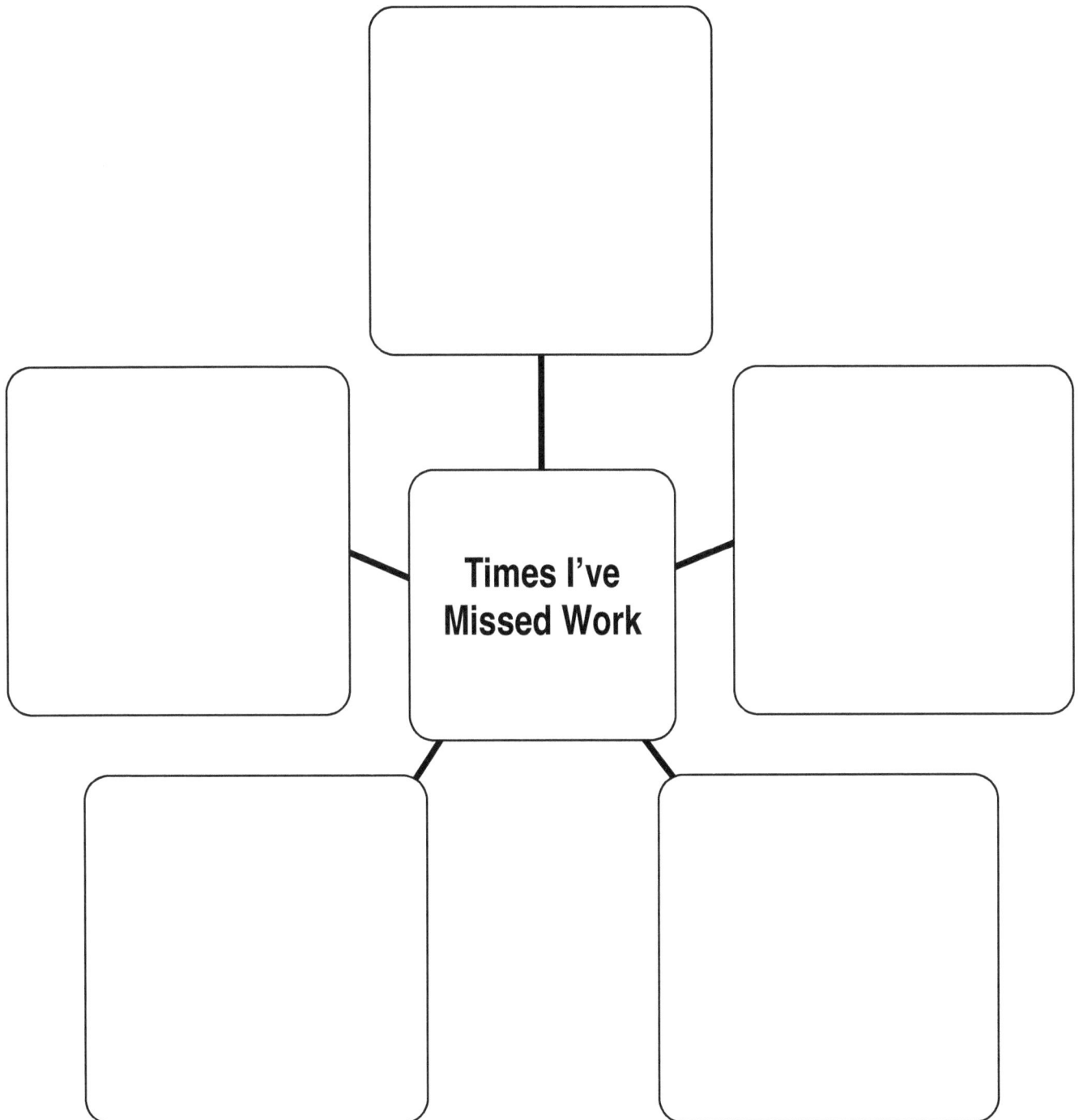

```
              ┌──────────┐
              │          │
              │          │
              │          │
              └────┬─────┘
┌──────────┐       │       ┌──────────┐
│          │   ┌───┴────┐  │          │
│          │───│Times I've│──│          │
│          │   │Missed Work│ │          │
└──────────┘   └──┬────┬──┘  └──────────┘
          ┌───────┘    └───────┐
     ┌────────┐          ┌────────┐
     │        │          │        │
     │        │          │        │
     └────────┘          └────────┘
```

Impacting Relationships

Excessive workouts start to impact the relationships of people addicted to exercise. When they spend so much time training that they miss a child's recital, rarely see their partner, or opt to stay at the gym instead of attending social get-togethers with friends, it could indicate an unhealthy relationship with exercise.

As with an eating disorder or substance abuse problem, people addicted to exercise tend to withdraw and isolate themselves from their friends and family to continue unhealthy behaviors.

Below, identify the times your exercising has impacted your relationships.

Times I Withdrew or Isolated Myself with Exercise	Why I Withdrew or Isolated Myself	How It Has Affected My Relationship with Others (USE NAME CODES)
Example: I stay at the gym rather than go home after work.	We constantly fight about finances and my not being at home.	MBW and I are growing apart.

It seems essential, in relationships and all tasks, that we concentrate
only on what is most significant and important.
~ Soren Kierkegaard

© 2023 WHOLE PERSON ASSOCIATES, 101 WEST 2ND STREET, SUITE 203, DULUTH MN 55802 • 800-247-6789 • WHOLEPERSON.COM

Are Necessary Tasks Happening?

Overexercising isn't a good idea for many reasons. It takes away much-needed time for regular tasks (laundry, cleaning the house, yard work, schoolwork, taking proper care of children), and it's also physically unhealthy.

Below, identify the tasks you are not getting done because you overexercise.

Tasks Not Completed:	Why Am I Unable to Complete My Tasks?	How Can I Change My Behav-ior?
Example: I am always late in pay-ing bills.	*I don't have time between workouts.*	*I can set aside time one night a week to pay bills.*

Tips for Managing Your Time Better:
- Before you begin each day, list urgent tasks that must be completed on specific days, while exercising can be carried over to the next day.
- Schedule essential tasks to ensure that they get completed.
- When you have a task, set a realistic deadline and stick to it.
- Do not let exercising interfere with important tasks.

Priorities Suffer

When you spend all your time exercising, other priorities suffer. (Example: due to overexercising, you missed an important work deadline, missed a child's volleyball game, or missed your 10th wedding anniversary.) It becomes a problem when you view and treat exercise as more significant than other priorities in your life.

Identify times when your priorities were not in order, and you missed something significant.

Areas of My Life	I Missed …	What I Was Doing Instead
Family		
Friends		
Work/Volunteer		
School		
Community		
Religious/Spiritual		
Other		

I'd like to be remembered as one who kept my priorities in the right order.
~ S. Truett Cathy

© 2023 WHOLE PERSON ASSOCIATES, 101 WEST 2ND STREET, SUITE 203, DULUTH MN 55802 • 800-247-6789 • WHOLEPERSON.COM

Exercise Burnout

Exercise burnout is a state of emotional, physical, and mental exhaustion caused by excessive and prolonged exercise. It occurs when you feel overwhelmed, emotionally drained, and unable to meet the constant demands of working out.

Below are ways your body will let you know you're headed for exercise burnout. Describe if and how each one affects you, how you noticed, and what you did (or could do) about it.

Signs of Exercise Burnout	How I Noticed This Sign	What I Did/Could Do
Example: *Decreased Performance*	*I could not swim as far or as long as I did in the past.*	*I started resting more between my workouts. I even took entire days off without swimming.*
Decreased Performance		
Disinterest in Working Out		
Changes in Mood		
Can't Recover as Quickly		
Extreme Fatigue		
Inability to Sleep		
Stopped Eating		
Overeating		

Can Too Much Exercise
Cause Physical Health Problems?

Even though regular exercise is healthy and strengthens the muscles and bones, too much physical activity increases the risk of physical and emotional issues. People with existing injuries risk aggravating their injuries and increasing the duration of recovery time.

Some examples of health issues caused by excessive exercise are below. Place a check before the physical problems you have experienced and describe your issue.

☐ **Muscle, tendon, ligament, sprain, back, knee: soreness or tenderness.**

_____

_____

_____

☐ **Gastrointestinal disturbances.**

_____

_____

_____

☐ **Decreased ability to ward off infection.**

_____

_____

_____

☐ **Elevated heart rate.**

_____

_____

_____

☐ **Elevated blood pressure.**

_____

_____

_____

☐ **Headaches.**

_____

_____

© 2023 WHOLE PERSON ASSOCIATES, 101 WEST 2ND STREET, SUITE 203, DULUTH MN 55802 • 800-247-6789 • WHOLEPERSON.COM

Can Too Much Exercise
Cause Emotional Health Problems?

Some emotional health issues that may be caused by excessive exercise are below.

Place a check in front of the problems you have experienced and describe your issue.

☐ **Diminished appetite or gained weight.**

_____

_____

_____

☐ **Anxiety.**

_____

_____

_____

☐ **Depression.**

_____

_____

_____

☐ **Compulsive need to exercise.**

_____

_____

_____

☐ **Exhaustion, constant fatigue, trouble sleeping.**

_____

_____

_____

☐ **Mood swings.**

_____

_____

_____

☐ **Disinterested in your workouts but feel like you can't take a break.**

_____

_____

_____

How Well Are You Sleeping?

Most people think that exercise can help people sleep. The opposite is often true. People who overexercise tend to experience sleep issues. Working out too close to bedtime can cause insomnia because your adrenaline is high, your brain is active, and it's difficult to wind down.

In the hexagrams below, identify the times you have had trouble sleeping, and explore what you were doing before going to bed.

When I Had Trouble Sleeping

© 2023 WHOLE PERSON ASSOCIATES, 101 WEST 2ND STREET, SUITE 203, DULUTH MN 55802 • 800-247-6789 • WHOLEPERSON.COM

A Healthy Conception of Self

Read the following quotation and respond to the questions that follow it.

Yes, I talk about eating disorders and you know, excessive dieting and excessive exercising can be a sign of a mental illness ... but when we talk about eating disorders... the issue is not the food or the exercise, the issue is a lack of healthy conception of self. That is the issue.
~ Sophie Gregoire Trudeau

In what ways do you agree or disagree with this quotation?

_____

_____

_____

Describe your diet habits as either reasonable or excessive. Why do you think this is true?

_____

_____

_____

Describe your exercise as either reasonable or excessive. Why do you think this is true?

_____

_____

_____

In what ways do you believe your eating and exercise behaviors are linked to your self-concept?

_____

_____

_____

What steps are you taking to overcome your overexercise issue?

_____

_____

_____

Self-Esteem Issue?

Low self-esteem is characterized by a lack of confidence and feeling badly about oneself.

People who overexercise or become obsessed with exercising often have self-esteem issues.

On the line under each symptom of low self-esteem, place an X on the continuum of how much you relate to the statement. On the dotted line below each one, write why you rated yourself that way. Be HONEST!

I hate the way I look.

0 (Not Like Me)   5 (Somewhat Like Me)   10 (Much Like Me)

I want a better body.

0 (Not Like Me)   5 (Somewhat Like Me)   10 (Much Like Me)

I must exercise to feel good about myself.

0 (Not Like Me)   5 (Somewhat Like Me)   10 (Much Like Me)

I compare my body to that of others.

0 (Not Like Me)   5 (Somewhat Like Me)   10 (Much Like Me)

I don't feel fulfilled unless I am working out.

0 (Not Like Me)   5 (Somewhat Like Me)   10 (Much Like Me)

I'm not good at anything else but training.

0 (Not Like Me)   5 (Somewhat Like Me)   10 (Much Like Me)

HIGHER SCORES (Much Like Me) on many of the statements indicate that you probably have an exercise addiction.

MEDIUM SCORES (Somewhat Like Me) other than getting a zero indicate a possible exercise addiction problem.

LOWER SCORES (Not Like Me) suggest that you are not experiencing many signs of an exercise problem.

© 2023 WHOLE PERSON ASSOCIATES, 101 WEST 2ND STREET, SUITE 203, DULUTH MN 55802 · 800-247-6789 · WHOLEPERSON.COM

Quotes about Problem Behavior

On the lines that follow each of the quotes, describe what the quote means to you and how it applies to YOUR life.

For me, it's all about balancing your priorities.
~ Gauri Khan

_____

_____

To me, self-esteem is not self-love. It is self-acknowledgment,
as in recognizing and accepting who you are.
~ Amity Gaige

_____

_____

Value your friendship. Value your relationships.
~ Barbara Bush

_____

_____

Action expresses priorities.
~ Mahatma Gandhi

_____

_____

Daily movement and exercise are a good thing, but it's possible to overdo it and
actually get in the way of your fitness goals, doing more harm than good to your body.
~ Alena Luciani, M.S., C.S.C.S.

_____

_____

Which quote especially speaks to you and your excessive exercise and why?

_____

_____

_____

_____

© 2023 WHOLE PERSON ASSOCIATES, 101 WEST 2ND STREET, SUITE 203, DULUTH MN 55802 • 800-247-6789 • WHOLEPERSON.COM

Exercise

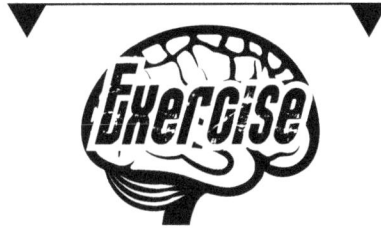

A Balanced Lifestyle

Name _____

Date _____

© 2023 WHOLE PERSON ASSOCIATES, 101 WEST 2ND STREET, SUITE 203, DULUTH MN 55802 • 800-247-6789 • WHOLEPERSON.COM

© 2023 WHOLE PERSON ASSOCIATES, 101 WEST 2ND STREET, SUITE 203, DULUTH MN 55802 • 800-247-6789 • WHOLEPERSON.COM

A Balanced Lifestyle Assessment
Introduction and Directions

People addicted to exercise need help to live a balanced lifestyle. They spend all their time focusing on working out and have little time left for sleep, rest, family, friends, social activities, work, and everyday activities. *The Balanced Lifestyle Assessment* is designed to help people evaluate how well they balance exercise with the rest of their life.

Read each statement and add a check mark in the box if the statement is descriptive of your exercising routines.

In the following example, the person completing the assessment checked two of the three exercise behaviors that are true for them:

When it comes to exercising and working out ...

☐ I believe in quantity, not quality.

☑ I often overexercise.

☐ I do not take a rest, even though I probably need to.

This is not a test. Since there are no right or wrong answers, do not spend too much time thinking about them. Be sure to respond to every statement.

BE HONEST!

If you choose, no one else needs to see the results.

(Turn to the next page and begin.)

A Balanced Lifestyle Assessment

Name _____ Date _____

This will only be accurate if you respond honestly. No one else needs to see this if you choose.

When it comes to exercising and working out …

☐ I believe in quantity, not quality.

☐ I often overexercise.

☐ I do not take a rest, even though I probably need to.

☐ I reward myself by doing more exercise.

☐ I don't listen to my body when it says it is time to stop.

☐ I have a reasonable routine but do not usually stick to it.

☐ I exercise when I am stressed.

☐ I don't believe that rest is very important.

☐ I ignore my body's signs saying I need a day of rest.

☐ I love exercising and resent being told it's too much.

☐ I do not feel the need to rest when I am in the middle of exercising.

☐ I think that resting is the same as laziness.

☐ I keep exercising even when my muscles are sore.

☐ I think that gentler forms of exercise are useless for me at this stage.

☐ I exercise even if I'm injured.

Number of items checked = _____

Go to the next page for scoring assessment results,
profile interpretation, and individual description.

© 2023 WHOLE PERSON ASSOCIATES, 101 WEST 2ND STREET, SUITE 203, DULUTH MN 55802 • 800-247-6789 • WHOLEPERSON.COM

A Balanced Lifestyle Assessment

Scoring Directions and Profile Interpretation

A Balanced Lifestyle Assessment that you just completed is designed to measure the extent to which you are aware of your body's capability to exercise in a healthy, balanced way.

***Count the number of items you checked and
place that number on the bottom line of the assessment.
Transfer that total to this space below:***

A Balanced Lifestyle TOTAL   =   _____

Assessment Profile Interpretation

The HIGHER your score on the Balanced Lifestyle Assessment, the more significant the extent of your addiction to exercise.

What surprises you about your score?

_____

_____

_____

What is one step you can immediately take to reduce your excessive exercise?

_____

_____

_____

Gentle Forms of Exercise

Exercising is valuable! We live in a society where everyone is loudly proclaiming the health benefits of exercise: It can control weight, combat health conditions, improve moods, promote good sleep, and it can be fun! However, it IS possible to overdo it, which can compromise your results. It's important to note that rest and gentler forms of movement are sometimes the healthiest choice.

Place a checkmark in the boxes by the exercises below that you have tried.
Place a checkmark in the boxes by those exercises you would be willing to try.

Exercises I Have Tried	Exercises I Would Try
☐ Aerobics	☐ Aerobics
☐ Balancing exercise	☐ Balancing exercise
☐ Chair exercises	☐ Chair exercises
☐ Cycling	☐ Cycling
☐ Dancing	☐ Dancing
☐ Get off a bus or a car early and walk the rest of the way	☐ Get off a bus or a car early and walk the rest of the way
☐ Golf or miniature golf	☐ Golf or miniature golf
☐ Hiking	☐ Hiking
☐ Ice skating	☐ Ice skating
☐ Isometrics	☐ Isometrics
☐ Pilates	☐ Pilates
☐ Plant a garden	☐ Plant a garden
☐ Push-ups	☐ Push-ups
☐ Qi Gong	☐ Qi Gong
☐ Rollerblading	☐ Rollerblading
☐ Sitting exercises	☐ Sitting exercises
☐ Stretching	☐ Stretching
☐ Swimming	☐ Swimming
☐ Tai Chi	☐ Tai Chi
☐ Walking	☐ Walking
☐ Water Exercise	☐ Water Exercise
☐ Weed pulling	☐ Weed pulling
☐ Weight lift with heavy cans	☐ Weight lift with heavy cans
☐ Yoga	☐ Yoga
☐ Zumba	☐ Zumba

© 2023 WHOLE PERSON ASSOCIATES, 101 WEST 2ND STREET, SUITE 203, DULUTH MN 55802 • 800-247-6789 • WHOLEPERSON.COM

Finding Your Own Balance

Knowing why you need exercise *(safe, healthy workout)*, rest *(sleeping and letting your body recuperate)*, and relaxation *(engaging in relaxing activities by yourself, with friends, or with family members)* is enlightening. Incorporating them into your life in a way that works well for you is a big deal! Adding all three of the above aspects into a healthy lifestyle is important for people who tend to overexercise.

Below, list the activities you ordinarily do and how long you spend on them daily.

Aspects of a Healthy Lifestyle	Activities (Write, Draw, or Doodle)	How Long I Spend on This Task Each Day
Exercise		
Rest		
Relaxation		

I think fitness is important. I think a healthy lifestyle is important. I think putting positive energy out there is important and just staying connected with the people.
~ LL Cool J

Regulate Your Sleep

Sleep is a critical component of a healthy lifestyle. People addicted to exercise often find that their minds or bodies are out of balance. When this occurs, people need to reflect on how much sleep they are getting. While 7-9 hours each night is recommended, most experts suggest you try to be consistent about when you go to bed and when you wake up each day. Consistency in your sleeping patterns will help ensure that you will get the most out of your rest and promote your health and well-being.

Below, track your sleep pattern each night for at least one week.

Days of the Week	Time I Went to Sleep	Time I Woke Up	How I Slept
Example: Monday	*1:00 am*	*6:30 am*	*I did not sleep well. I was up multiple times with sore calf muscles!*
Monday			
Tuesday			
Wednesday			
Thursday			
Friday			
Saturday			
Sunday			

© 2023 WHOLE PERSON ASSOCIATES, 101 WEST 2ND STREET, SUITE 203, DULUTH MN 55802 • 800-247-6789 • WHOLEPERSON.COM

Sleeping Well

Part of taking good care of yourself includes getting a good night's sleep. However, when people excessively exercise, it's tempting to keep working out late into the evening. Besides not exercising before going to bed, sleep experts offer a variety of suggestions designed to help people improve their sleep hygiene.

Below, check the actions you take and explain how you do them.

Before I go to bed ...

☐ I use relaxation techniques. _____

☐ I do deep breathing exercises. _____

☐ I relax my muscles progressively._____

☐ I do a quick meditation session. _____

☐ I make sure my bedroom is dark._____

☐ I set the temperature to be comfortable for me. _____

☐ I power down electronic devices and do not use them in bed._____

☐ I sleep on a comfortable mattress and with a comfy pillow._____

☐ I stay hydrated by drinking plenty of water throughout the day._____

☐ I avoid alcohol close to bedtime._____

☐ I do not consume caffeine late in the day. _____

☐ I try to stick to a sleep schedule._____

☐ I work on limiting daytime naps. _____

☐ I try not to worry when I am going to sleep. _____

Look over your responses. How successful have you been when it comes to sleep habits?

_____

_____

What can you do better?_____

_____

Home-Based Workout

People addicted to exercise often choose the most high-intensity workout available to them. One way to reduce overexercising is to exercise around the house. Some ways to do this include gardening, cutting grass, washing household windows, walking the stairs, doing household chores, etc. This way, you can choose to completely skip your workout and stay active overall during the day.

In the spaces below, identify several ways to skip a workout and exercise at home.

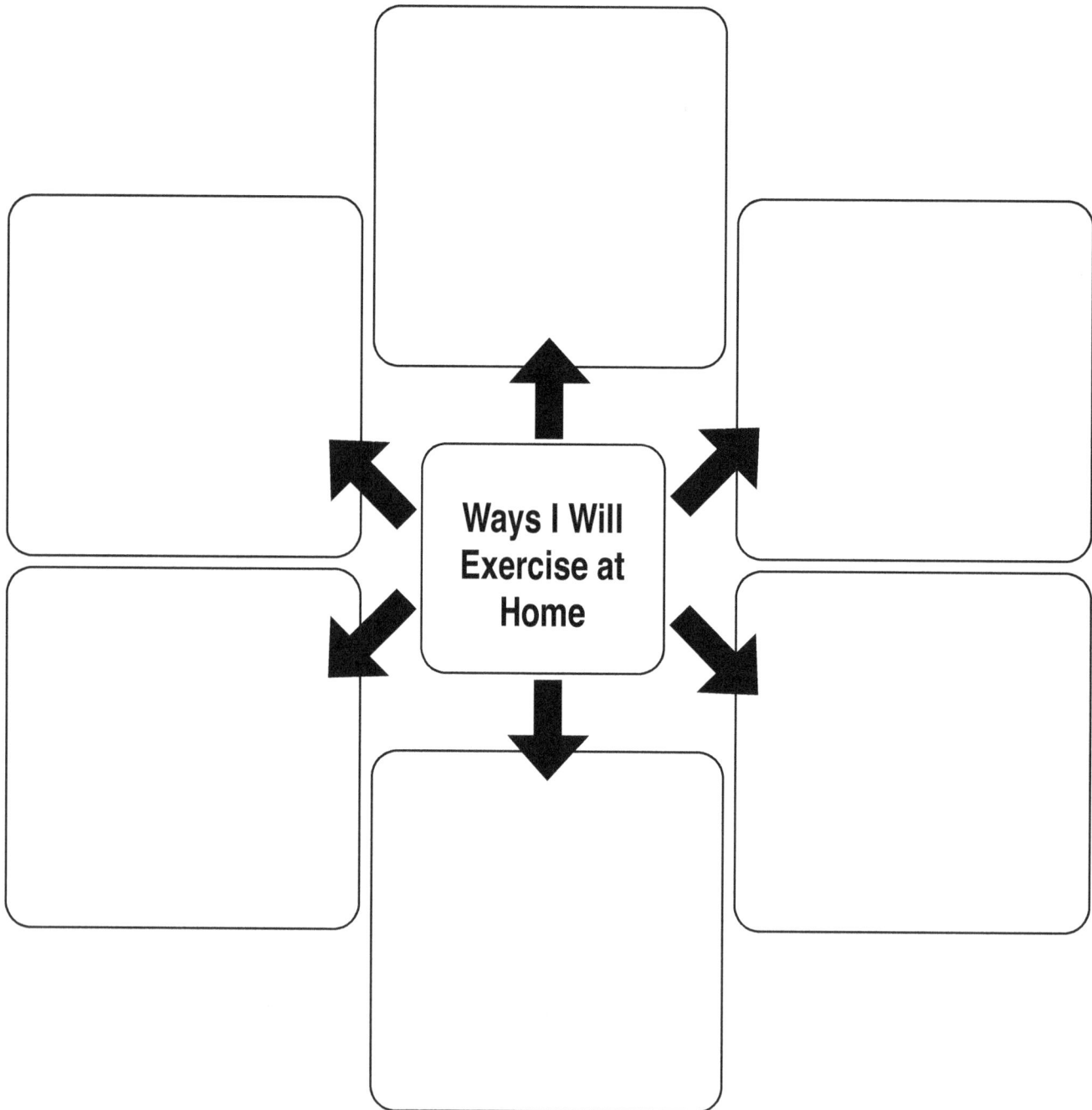

Ways I Will Exercise at Home

Keep an Exercise Journal

It is important to reflect on your day with an exercise journal by writing how much and how you exercised. This journal can help you plan your workout and rest days and help you keep track and stick to a balanced routine. Your journal can be something you keep in a little notebook, three-ring binder, or a downloaded fitness app. You can track your progress, how your body feels during and after exercising, and awareness of when you're fatigued and need rest.

Days of the Week	Notes
Monday	
Tuesday	
Wednesday	
Thursday	
Friday	
Saturday	
Sunday	

Reproduce this form to journal for future weeks.

Mix It Up

Many people addicted to exercise concentrate on one high-intensity workout mode. If they are exercising excessively, they need to keep their workouts balanced. Someone can be an avid runner, engage in Pilates, and lift weights. Mixing up training can give a person resistance and endurance in their weekly schedule, which helps keep their mind and body healthy.

In the circles below, identify multiple ways you can engage in training to mix things up.

Ways I Will Mix It Up

© 2023 WHOLE PERSON ASSOCIATES, 101 WEST 2ND STREET, SUITE 203, DULUTH MN 55802 • 800-247-6789 • WHOLEPERSON.COM

How to Write an Exercise Schedule

An exercise schedule is a great tool to use when you're trying to exercise without neglecting personal obligations. You can schedule different days/hours of exercise, work, rest, home obligations, family time, paying bills, television, games, sports, outdoor chores, etc. An exercise schedule can help you plan exactly how much time you will dedicate to training, obligations, and other fun things in your life!

Step 1: Start your schedule by writing in all the workouts you will do during the week. Be specific with each date and time.

Step 2: Pencil in your rest days and times. After completing your exercise schedule, you can look at what day or two is the best for rest. Make sure to pencil this in – it may change as your week progresses. Try to be flexible with your rest day, as you may feel differently than expected during your week. You may have something pop up to push back workouts or feel more tired or sore than anticipated.

TIPS FOR HEALTHY WORKOUTS:

- The sequence in which you plan light days of exercise, heavy days of exercise, and rest days is essential.

- In general, you want to alternate days of more work or intense exercise with days of rest or light-intensity exercise.

- If you have an injury or a medical condition, consult your doctor or an exercise therapist for help designing a fitness program that gradually improves your range of motion, strength, and endurance.

- Schedule time to exercise as you would any other appointment. Plan to watch your favorite show while walking on the treadmill, read while riding a stationary bike, or go for a walk during work downtime.

- Include many different activities. Cross-training can make exercising more fun.

- Allow plenty of time for rest and recovery.

- Break things up if you can. You don't have to do all your exercise at once, so you can weave in activities throughout your day. Exercising in short sessions a few times a day may fit your schedule better than a single session.

- Use a lifestyle approach. Your workout routine might include walking, bicycling, rowing, hiking with your family, or ballroom dancing.

- Listen to your body. Take a break if you feel pain, shortness of breath, dizziness, or nausea. You may be pushing yourself too hard.

- Be flexible, and don't stick to your workout schedule rigidly. If you're not feeling well, give yourself permission to take a day or two off.

My Exercise Schedule

Days of the Week	Exercise Work Out Time and Activities	Rest and Restoration Time and Activities
Example: Monday	6:15 am – Run for 30 minutes 7:15 am – Weight lift for 60 minutes Noon – lunchtime – Martial arts training for 60 minutes	5 pm – Play with children for 20 minutes 6 pm –Watch TV with family for a few hours 10 pm – Read for 30 minutes before bedtime
Monday		
Tuesday		
Wednesday		
Thursday		
Friday		
Saturday		
Sunday		

If we could give every individual the right amount of nourishment and exercise, not too little and not too much, we would have found the safest way to health.
~ Hippocrates

© 2023 WHOLE PERSON ASSOCIATES, 101 WEST 2ND STREET, SUITE 203, DULUTH MN 55802 • 800-247-6789 • WHOLEPERSON.COM

Healthy Re-Engagement

People addicted to exercise need healthy substitutes when reducing their workout behavior. These healthy substitutes can help structure time, distract from exercising, and enhance self-esteem. Some examples of these worthwhile activities include writing, painting, playing chess, singing, gardening, volunteering, etc.

What are four healthy substitutes for your excessive exercise behavior? Write about them, draw them, or doodle them in the spaces below.

1.	2.
3.	**4.**

Make Time Just For You

People who are addicted to exercise work out so much and so often that they do not make time to take care of themselves in other ways. They put exercise before everything else, including themselves.

Below, identify some of the things you can do just for yourself. These might include reading a good mystery, taking a nap, or walking the dog (or a neighbor's dog).

Just For Me

© 2023 WHOLE PERSON ASSOCIATES, 101 WEST 2ND STREET, SUITE 203, DULUTH MN 55802 • 800-247-6789 • WHOLEPERSON.COM

Making Small Changes

A positive attitude is critical in overcoming a behavioral addiction. When people realize that they are overexercising, they need to take on a positive attitude when making small changes in their approach to living a healthier lifestyle.

Some ways to make small changes and remain positive are listed below. Write about how you can (and will) make small changes in your exercise routine.

Change to different forms of exercise.
Revise current workout regimes.
Add days of rest.
Avoid too many trips to the gym or the place where you work out.
Work on keeping a positive attitude.

The above changes would benefit anyone who wants to reduce their addiction to exercise and enjoy a happier, healthier lifestyle.

How do you think these small changes would affect you and your relationships?

_____

_____

_____

Rest and Restore

For people who overexercise, an important rule is to listen to what your body is telling you...
REST and RESTORE!

If your body needs a day off, take it. Your body has ways of telling you that you're overdoing your training. If you feel strained, exhausted, fatigued, or sick, that's a sign that it just might be time to take a step back and skip that day's workout. Think about when your body has talked to you.

Identify the ways your body tells you to stop and rest, whether you listen or not, and the end results.

How My Body Tells Me to Rest	How I Rest and Restore	End Result
Example: When I sleep longer than usual, my body is telling me I need to rest and restore.	*I take the day off from exercising after work, come home, relax, and hang out with family.*	*By bedtime, I feel my body getting stronger and ready to exercise the next day.*

Rest until you feel like playing, then play until you feel like resting, period.
Never do anything else.
~ Martha Beck

© 2023 WHOLE PERSON ASSOCIATES, 101 WEST 2ND STREET, SUITE 203, DULUTH MN 55802 • 800-247-6789 • WHOLEPERSON.COM

Signs that You Need a Rest Day

People who are addicted to exercise do not want to take days off to rest. If you notice any of the following signs, it might be time to take a break!

On the line under each sign, place an X on the continuum of how much you relate to the statement. On the dotted line below each one, write why you rated yourself that way. BE HONEST!

After my workout I ...

I had sore muscles.

0 (Stopped Exercising)   5 (Slowed Down)   10 (Kept Exercising)

I was fatigued.

0 (Stopped Exercising)   5 (Slowed Down)   10 (Kept Exercising)

I didn't feel like exercising at all.

0 (Stopped Exercising)   5 (Slowed Down)   10 (Kept Exercising)

I experienced emotional changes.

0 (Stopped Exercising)   5 (Slowed Down)   10 (Kept Exercising)

I have not been sleeping well.

0 (Stopped Exercising)   5 (Slowed Down)   10 (Kept Exercising)

I did not see increased performance.

0 (Stopped Exercising)   5 (Slowed Down)   10 (Kept Exercising)

KEPT EXERCISING scores on statements indicate that you definitely need to take rest days.

SLOWED DOWN scores other than getting a 0 can mean that you are cutting when you need to.

STOPPED EXERCISING suggests that you seem to be doing the right thing about resting, but it does indicate that you need to be careful.

Ways I Overexercise

It is essential for people who overexercise to look at the specific struggles they have with exercise and increase their insight into how exercise addiction manifests itself.

For the various ways people overtrain listed below, write about the ones that apply to you and how you can limit this excessive exercise in the future.

Ways I Overtrain	Effect It Has on Me	How I Can Limit Training
Example: Extending workouts.	*I get so tired I cannot sleep at night.*	*Set and carry a stopwatch and quit when the alarm goes off.*
Extending Workouts		
Not Resting or Taking Breaks		
Doing Multiple Sessions Each Day		
Exercising When I'm Sick or Injured		
Obsessing About Exercising		
Other		

Respect your efforts, respect yourself. Self-respect leads to self-discipline. When you have both firmly under your belt, that's real power.
~ Clint Eastwood

© 2023 WHOLE PERSON ASSOCIATES, 101 WEST 2ND STREET, SUITE 203, DULUTH MN 55802 • 800-247-6789 • WHOLEPERSON.COM

Quotes About a Healthy Lifestyle

On the lines that follow each of the quotes, describe what the quote means to you and how it applies to Your life.

Making small changes every week over a few months will result in huge changes.
~ Ella Woodward

_____

_____

We all have dreams. But in order to make dreams come into reality, it takes an awful lot of determination, dedication, self-discipline, and effort.
~ Jesse Owens

_____

_____

Self-care equals success. You're going to be more successful if you take care of yourself and you're healthy.
~ Beth Behrs

_____

_____

Good things come to those that sweat!
~ Anonymous

_____

_____

Which quote especially speaks to you about a healthy lifestyle? Why?

_____

_____

_____

_____

_____

_____

_____

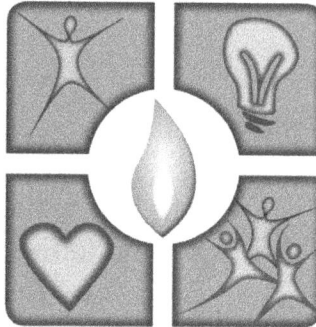

WholePerson

Whole Person Associates is the leading publisher of training resources for professionals who empower people to create and maintain healthy lifestyles. Our creative resources will help you work effectively with your clients in the areas of stress management, wellness promotion, mental health, and life skills.

Please visit us at our website: **WholePerson.com**. You can check out our entire line of products, place an order, request our print catalog, and sign up for our monthly special notifications.

Whole Person Associates
800-247-6789
Books@WholePerson.com

www.ingramcontent.com/pod-product-compliance
Lightning Source LLC
Chambersburg PA
CBHW082359270326
41935CB00013B/1683